Have You Been Outside Today?

108 things you can do to get out of a funk.

Rae-Anne

About The Author

Rae-Anne is a speaker, coach, writer and mental health educator. Although not formally diagnosed until the age of 47, she has lived with depression and anxiety for most of her adult life. Rae-Anne lives in Adelaide, Australia with her husband Shanton. She has two adult children who make her proud every day and two gorgeous grandchildren. When she's not in Bali (she goes there a lot) she can usually be found drinking tea, talking too loud and buying more books than she can ever read.

You can find her at www.rae-anne.com.au and www.transpiral.com.au

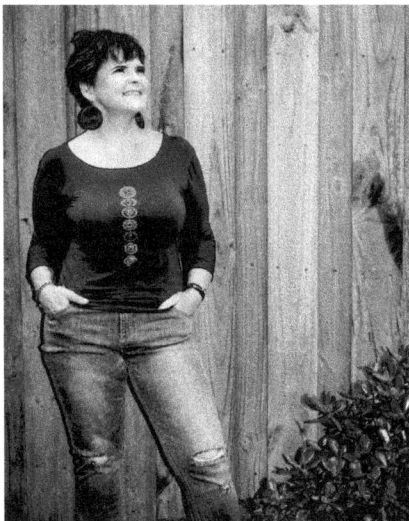

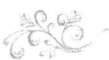 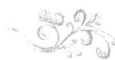

For my mum, who taught
me that anything is possible.

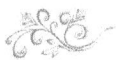 Have you been outside today?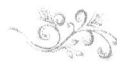

Contents

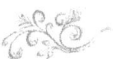

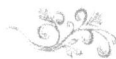

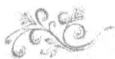

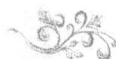

Foreword

"Have you been outside today?" I read. At first this question strikes me as absurd and I wave a dismissive hand at the computer screen.

Well, of course I... hang on; have I?

If you're like me, you probably have a lot on your plate. A fulfilling but demanding work schedule, friends and family who squeeze like Tetris blocks into the gaps in your calendar, and maybe you're juggling study commitments too.

If you're like me, perhaps you experience great difficulty in saying "no". You'll take on that extra task, be on "just one more" committee, stay out with that friend who wants some company even though yesterday you swore that tonight would be your "alone time". And maybe, just maybe, you have agreed to write a foreword to a book with absolutely no idea of how to do it.

This is not a bad thing. After all, we do all of these things out of love. Love for our friends, our jobs, our families. We are so busy loving everyone, committing to everything that we not only forget to love and commit to ourselves, the idea becomes laughable. And yet, when we board an aeroplane,

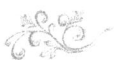

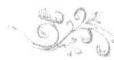

Have you been outside today?

we do not laugh when the instructional video tells us that we should put on our own oxygen mask before helping others.

I lived a life diminished, squandered, and ravished by depression and anxiety for many years. Just as it took a village to raise me, it took a village to raise me up from the depths of poor mental health. A medley of pills, family, friends, support groups, and psychologist and psychiatrist appointments, helped me slowly, ever so slowly, to imagine something that looked vaguely like a life. And as I started to get better, my psychologist and I began to talk about how I would maintain my new-found well-being. And this is when – and I hope you'll forgive both the crudeness and the slight irony of what I am about to say – I began to believe that my psychologist had gone a little mad.

She talked to me of meditation, breathing, sleeping eight hours a night, eating well, exercising, reading books, and spending time in nature. This simply did not make sense to me. After all, the medication, the support groups, the appointments had all been so regimented, so "official" in their status as treatment. How could it be that the rest of the solution lay in something so... ordinary?

Besides, I *didn't have time* for all that stuff. Now that I was well again, I needed to find a career, my own home, relationships. In short, now that I had a life, I needed to live it.

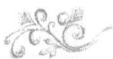

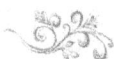

Well, this book is for people who don't have time. It artfully breaks the often maligned language of self-care down into practical, achievable, and even enjoyable activities. It reminds us to put on our own oxygen mask. It teaches us that caring for ourselves is the first step to being able to properly care for others, and to achieve all that we need to. And, perhaps most importantly, it reminds us that self-care is not a luxury but a responsibility; a debt that we owe to ourselves and everyone who loves us. The use of concise, clear language shows something that is at once comforting and extremely irritating: that we have known what to do all along! So next time you think you don't have time for one of the activities in this book, or for something else that helps you, ask yourself: *Do I have time to become unwell? Do I have time to be unhappy?*

Rae-Anne, thank you for your passion, and your compassion. Thank you for being such a clear, strong, yet gentle voice calling us back from our busy lives. And to the readers, thank you for supporting local writers, and thank you for supporting yourselves.

With love,

Kelly Vincent
Dignity Party MLC, South Australian Parliament

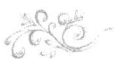

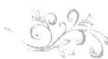

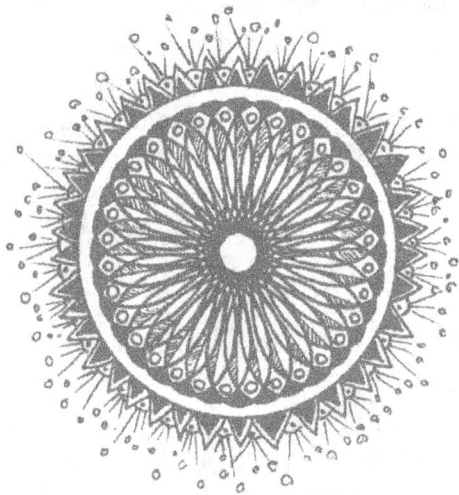

Introduction

The idea for this book came to me as I was writing a chapter for my book *How I learnt to love my bum and other lessons from Africa*. I began writing the chapter on corruption and before long I found myself so worked up that I didn't know what to do with my body or mind.

It reminded me of those serious funk days, those days where all I want to do is lie on the couch, eat chocolate and watch nonsense on TV while mindlessly scrolling through Facebook, because I couldn't think of anything else to do.

I started writing a list of things I find helpful during those times, with the idea that it might become a deck of cards. I then had the idea to create it as a little e-book, and I thought it would be a nice piece to share with people. I invited friends to include stories of experiences they've had with funk days, whether or not they have been diagnosed with a mental illness, and the things they have found helpful to overcome them. Some shared hints and tips; others opened their lives and bared their souls. Their stories are real, raw, courageous and honest.

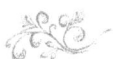

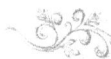

I showed a few friends and they loved it. They said they needed it. They said they wanted to carry it with them at all times.

The book has grown into so much more than a book. It's become a community. It's a community that has brought people together to realise that none of us is alone. Ever.

I'm so excited and honoured to have been part of this coming together of people willing to share their lives, their darkest and brightest times and their healing as a result of these moments.

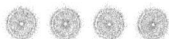

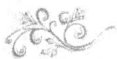

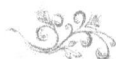

Some days everything just seems to suck.

We've all had those awful days where life just seems to be one giant vortex of yuck and funk. It's completely normal to have days like this. Some of us have them more often than others, but believe me when I tell you that we all have them.

Whether you've been diagnosed with depression, anxiety or any other mental illness – or not – this book is for you to use on those days when you need a little something to lift your mood. It's a reminder that this too will pass. And it will.

When I'm in a funk I find it hard to get my brain into a place where I can remember those things that make me feel better. It's also very difficult to get creative enough to make some up. But when I'm not in a funk, the thought of preparing myself better for the next one disappears, because of course I'm feeling fine! Why would I need to?

The suggestions in this book come from a wide range of resources. Some of them are mine. Some I've picked up over the years from family, friends and clients. People I know have shared others with me. I've also left some spaces for you to add your own, so you can build an even bigger list.

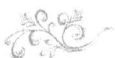

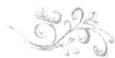

Please know that everything you're feeling is perfectly normal. If you've been feeling down for more than a week or two, or you feel that you need more than this book can provide, I've listed some helpful resources for you in the back.

May tomorrow be a better day.

Rae-Anne

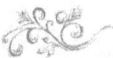 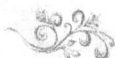

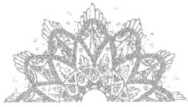

Character cannot be developed in ease
and quiet. Only through experience
of trial and suffering can the soul be
strengthened, ambition inspired, and
success achieved.

– Helen Keller

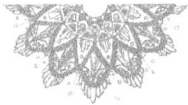

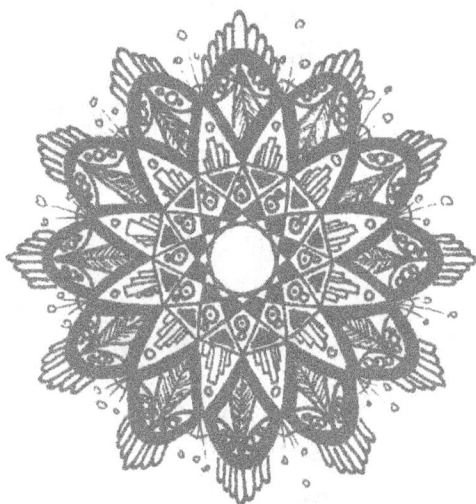

Chapter Two

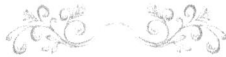

Things To Do At Home

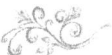 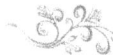

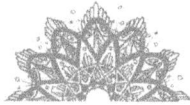

Maybe you have to know the darkness
before you can appreciate the light.

– Madeleine L'Engle

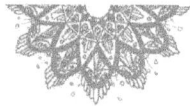

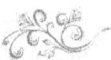

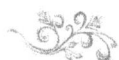

Go outside. Enjoy the warmth of the sun directly on your bare skin. Take three cleansing breaths of fresh air.

Ground yourself in nature. Take your shoes off and put your feet on the ground, whether grass, sand or dirt.

Take a shower. Notice the feeling of water against your skin, the scent of the soap, the sound of the water. Everything feels better after a shower.

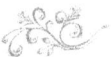 Have you been outside today?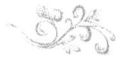

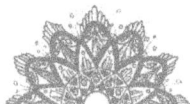

There are far, far better things ahead
than anything we leave behind.
— C. S. Lewis

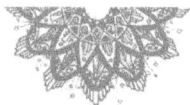

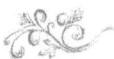 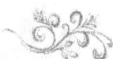

Put on music you love. Turn it up loud. Immerse yourself in the rhythm. Choose music that uplifts and inspires you. Rock, classical, reggae, it doesn't matter – whatever soothes your soul.

Create a funk day music playlist.

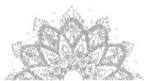

I get myself out of a funk by putting on noise cancelling earphones and blasting my favourite music with a cheeky glass of wine.

– Sara

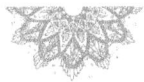

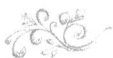 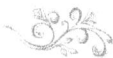

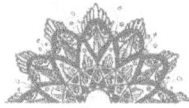

Sometimes you will never know the value
of a moment, until it becomes a memory.

– Dr Seuss

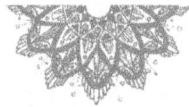

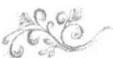 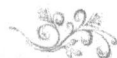

❀ Binge-watch your favourite TV show.

❀ Call a friend. Be sure to choose one who is a great listener, non-judgemental and always keeps it real.

❀ Meditate. Meditation has many proven benefits for mood. If you aren't sure how to meditate, download an app to get you started.

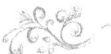

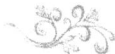

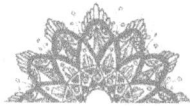

The greatest degree of inner tranquility comes from the development of love and compassion. The more we care for the happiness of others, the greater is our own sense of well-being.

— **Tenzin Gyatso**

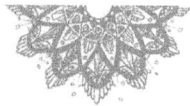

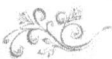

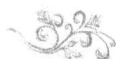

Take a deep bath. Light some candles, put on some gentle music, and soak and relax in the soothing water.

Light a candle, especially if it's one you've been saving for a special occasion. Every day is special and should be celebrated.

Practice gratitude. Even if you are feeling dreadful there are things to be thankful for. You can start with having food in your belly and a roof over your head. Taking time to notice things you are grateful for is a great way to shift your mood. Write them down. Try to list at least three. Do it again tomorrow, and try to make it a regular habit.

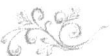 Have you been outside today?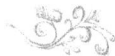

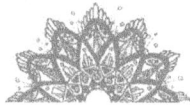

At least three times every day take
a moment and ask yourself: what is
really important? Have the wisdom and
the courage to build your life around
your answer.

– Lee Jampolsky

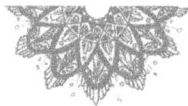

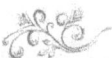

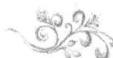

Wear clothes that make you feel confident. It takes as much time to put on nice clothes as it does to put on sweatpants. When you're in a funk, you will most likely want to wear the sweatpants. Fight the urge. The Look Good/Feel Better campaign was aimed at people living with cancer and chemotherapy; but you can learn something from it too.

Eat something beautiful. Buy the best you can afford of your favourite food, whether that's fruit, chocolate or cake. Make it spectacular and savour every single delicious mouthful.

Burn incense. Get your olfactory senses excited by the exotic scents that only incense can provide.

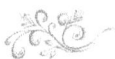

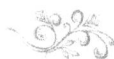

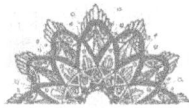

If you're going through Hell, keep going.

— Winston Churchill

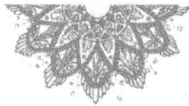

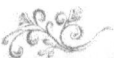

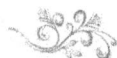

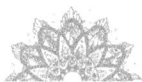 Declutter. Decluttering can be a very cathartic process. Get rid of clothes that you no longer wear. Clear out your cupboards. Throw out all the plastic containers in the kitchen without lids, and ditch those cups and plates with chips and cracks. Immerse yourself in the process.

Clean your windows as they are the eyes to the soul. The action of cleaning can often allow the mind to wander through all sorts of muck in order to get clarity. Another one is to tidy up a drawer. Seeing something nice and orderly without the unwanted things can lead to more tidying – but it will also help put things into perspective.

– Suzanne

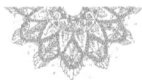

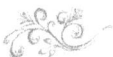 Have you been outside today?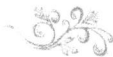

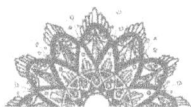

Start by doing what's necessary; then
do what's possible; and suddenly you are
doing the impossible.

– St. Francis of Assisi

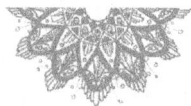

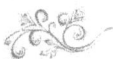

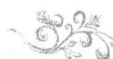

Garden. There is something special about being connected with the earth. Pull some weeds, tidy up a few things and maybe even get some new plants. If you have a small balcony or courtyard, create a small potted garden. Afterwards be sure to sit down with a nice cuppa and admire your handiwork.

Write. You could keep a journal, start a blog, or just doodle and scribble. Getting your thoughts onto paper is cathartic. Write like nobody is ever going to read it – your thoughts, feelings, dreams, and hopes. Whatever comes, let it flow. Just write it down.

Watch your favourite movie. Preferably not a tearjerker! Try to find one that's always guaranteed to give you a laugh.

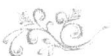

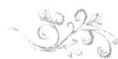

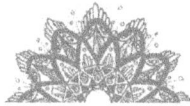

And the day came when the risk it took
to remain tight inside the bud was more
painful than the risk it took to blossom.

– Anais Nin

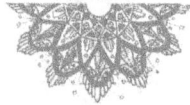

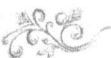 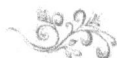

❋ Plan a holiday. Research has shown that there can be as much joy and fun in the planning as the actual trip. Look at photos of the places you'd love to see. Go to those places – even if only in your mind for today.

❋ Do nothing. Simply stop for a while, sit back, and take a few mindful breaths.

❋ Watch a funny cat/dog/human video on YouTube. You know the ones that you can't help but giggle at. Keep your favourites in a playlist for easy reference.

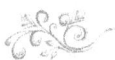

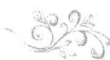

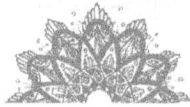

Every blade of grass has its angel that
bends over it and whispers, 'Grow, grow'.

– The Talmud

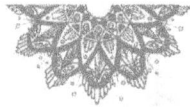

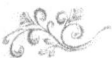 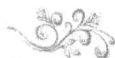

Pick some fresh flowers and put them in a vase by your bed.

Is it time for a new hairstyle? Browse different styles online and save a few for your next visit to the hairdresser.

Name how you are feeling. Naming our emotions tends to diffuse their impact and lessen the burden they create. Noticing and naming gives us the chance to take a step back and make choices about what to do with them.

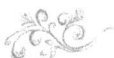 Have you been outside today?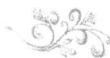

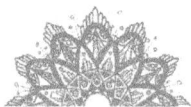

Even the darkest night will end and the
sun will rise.

— Victor Hugo

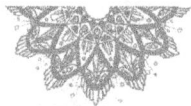

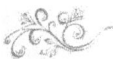 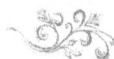

✤ Hug a furry friend. If you don't have one of your own, find someone who does.

✤ Hug a human friend. Research shows that hugging is extremely effective at healing sickness, disease, loneliness, depression, anxiety and stress.

✤ Buy a beautiful bouquet of flowers for yourself. You deserve it.

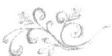

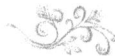

Have you been outside today?

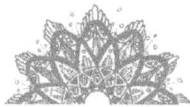

Our grand business is not to see what
lies dimly at a distance, but to do what
lies clearly at hand.

– Thomas Carlyle

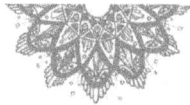

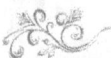

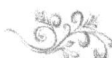

✺ Do a random act of kindness. Performing random acts of kindness helps boost your psychological health by activating the release of dopamine, the feel-good neurotransmitter in the brain, often referred to as a "helper's high". This is based on the theory that giving to others produces endorphins in the brain that mimic a morphine high. Simply being motivated by generosity can benefit you as much as it does those receiving your help.

✺ Write a gratitude letter. Gratitude is strongly and consistently associated with greater happiness. Gratitude helps people feel more positive emotions, relish good experiences, improve their health, deal with adversity and build strong relationships.

✺ Do you have a flow activity? Do that. People in flow also tend to feel cheerful, strong, active, concentrated, creative and satisfied. Self-esteem increases after a flow experience, and people who are in flow more often have higher self-esteem overall. (For more on flow, see resources at the back of this book.)

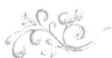

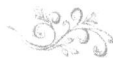

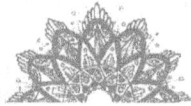

You have been assigned this mountain
to show others it can be moved."

– Unknown

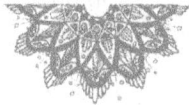

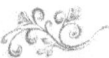 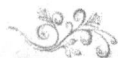

* Read a book. Find a super comfy place, curl up and immerse yourself in the story.

* Essential oils. Make or use a nourishing blend, use a diffuser or an oil burner and enjoy the healing aromas.

* Send a thank you card.

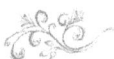 Have you been outside today?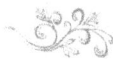

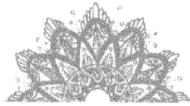

Your breathing is your greatest friend.
Return to it in all your trouble and your
will find comfort and guidance.

– Unknown

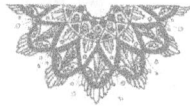

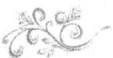 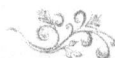

- Drink tea – any tea. Sit quietly and enjoy every warming mouthful.

- Drink a big glass of water. Recent studies have shown that even mild dehydration can influence mood, energy levels and the ability to think clearly.

- Check out some food porn. Get those creative juices flowing and plan your meals for the week.

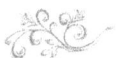
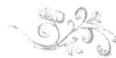

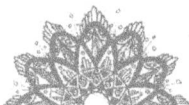

Sometimes we fall down because
there is something down there we are
supposed to find.

– Emily Joy Rosen

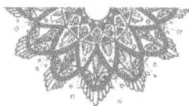

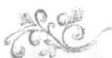

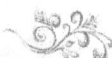

❀ Paint your nails. It may be a small thing, but it can make you feel pretty and give you a pick-me-up. Choose a bright happy colour.

❀ Clean the house. It may be like the last thing you feel like doing at first, so start small. Clean one thing. See if that inspires you to do more. The combined benefits of moving, feeling productive and having something at the end to admire, giving a sense of accomplishment, can be a great mood booster.

❀ Colouring. Adult colouring books are the new black. Grab one and make your inner child happy.

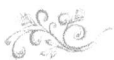

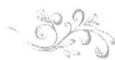

Have you been outside today?

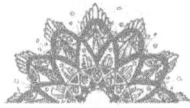

No grit, no pearl.

– Unknown

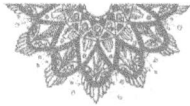

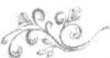 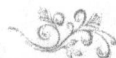

❋ Zentangle. If you don't know what this is, look it up online. Zentangles are mindful doodles. The Zentangle method is an easy-to-learn, relaxing and fun way to create beautiful images by drawing structured patterns.

❋ Make art. Any medium will do. Paint, sketch, sculpt, knit, sew, crochet, beading...create something.

❋ On a hot day, wash the car. Spray water in the air to form a rainbow to remind yourself that it takes a little rain and a little sun to create something that beautiful. A little negative and a little positive is needed to create the rainbow of life.

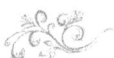

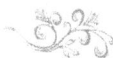

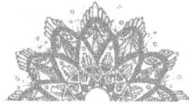

Nourishing yourself in a way that helps
you blossom in the direction you want
to go is attainable, and you are worth
the effort.

– Deborah Day

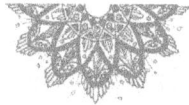

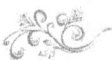 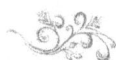

Stop and appreciate life just as it is. The first thing you did this morning was to take a breath, so be thankful for that. Some of us may see today's sunrise but not the sunset. Be present.

Sing. Sing loud. In the shower, in the car, in the lounge – it doesn't matter where or how your voice sounds, just sing!

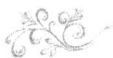

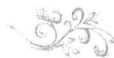

Do a jigsaw puzzle.

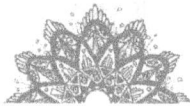

Life is all about balance. You don't
always need to be getting stuff done.
Sometimes it's perfectly OK and
absolutely necessary to shut down, kick
back, and do nothing.

— Lori Deschene

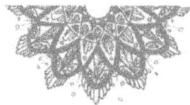

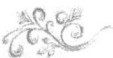

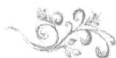

Play Patience. Play old school, with real cards.

Affirmations. Choose some affirmations that resonate with you and make you feel inspired. Say them over and over. Write them in places you will see them regularly such as the bathroom mirror and beside your bed. Fake it until you make it.

Cry. Let it all out. A good cry can be cleansing.

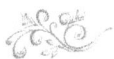 Have you been outside today?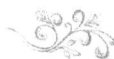

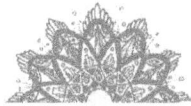

It's OK, you know, to be carried now and
then, strength too needs a rest.

– Tyler Knott Gregson

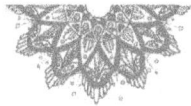

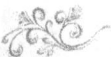

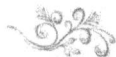

Sleep. Have a nap. Recharge those batteries. Sleep is healing and most of us don't get enough of it.

Bake. Make a cake, muffins or biscuits. Take a plate and give it to your neighbour.

Give yourself a facial. Do it at home – there is no need to go out and spend money to feel pampered.

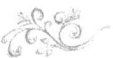 Have you been outside today?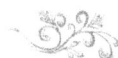

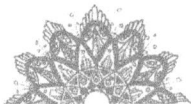

When life knocks you down, roll over, and
look at the stars.

– Unknown

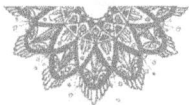

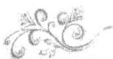 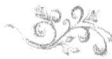

❀ Shave. Shave your face if you're a man, legs if you're a woman. Enjoy feeling refreshed and smooth!

❀ Make your bed. It's a great habit to develop every day if you don't do it already. Change the sheets while you are at it. A clean fresh bed is always a good thing.

❀ Set goals. Keep them SMART – that is, specific, measureable, achievable, realistic and time-based. Write them down and make a plan.

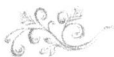

Have you been outside today?

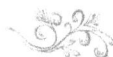

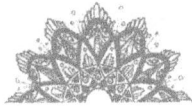

Think and wonder, wonder and think.

– Dr Seuss

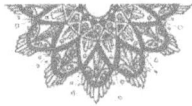

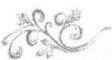 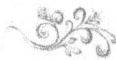

- Make a vision board. Put it somewhere you can see it every day.

- Play a board game.

- Drum. Studies have shown that repetitive drumming changes brain wave activity, inducing a state of calm and focused awareness.

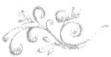 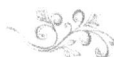

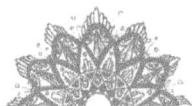

Let me not pray to be sheltered from dangers, but to be fearless in facing them. Let me not beg for the stilling of my pain, but for the heart to conquer it.

— **Rabindranath Tagore**

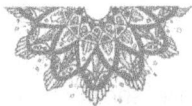

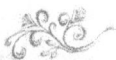

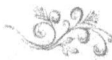

◈ Hug a tree.

◈ Hug yourself. One easy way to soothe and comfort yourself when you're feeling badly is to give yourself a gentle hug or caress, or simply put your hand on your heart and feel the warmth of your hand. It may feel awkward or embarrassing at first, but your body doesn't know that. It just responds to the physical gesture of warmth and care, just as a baby responds to being cuddled in its mother's arms.

◈ Learn something new. Developing new skills and achieving things lifts your mood. Research courses or workshops you can attend in your local area.

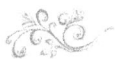

Have you been outside today?

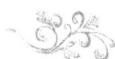

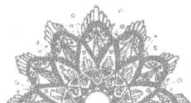

Promise me you'll always remember:
you're braver than you believe, and
stronger than you seem, and smarter
than you think.

– A.A. Milne

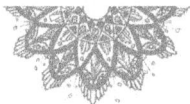

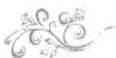 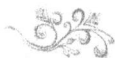

Computer games. Do you have a favourite? If so play that, or better yet, master a new one.

Comfort food. Treat yourself today. Whatever comfort food is for you: soft white bread and butter, cookie dough, chocolate, pizza, ice cream...

Do a crossword puzzle, word find or Sudoku puzzle.

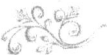 Have you been outside today?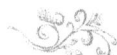

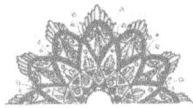

Self-care is taking the time to recover.
It's sabbaticals to clear your head
and chart your course. It's leaving. It's
investing. It's asking for more. It's being
protective and tender and limitlessly
compassionate with yourself.

– Danielle LaPorte

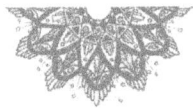

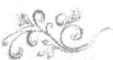

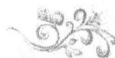

Blow bubbles. Embrace your fun-loving inner child.

Close your eyes for a few minutes. It's hard to truly comprehend how much time we spend with our eyes widened by the glaring light of our phones, TVs and computers. Not only is it physically straining, it's also mentally draining. Place your hands over your eyes for two minutes, and relish the time you have to sit still and be with yourself.

Lie on a blanket and look up at the clouds. Watch them float by in the sky and imagine them taking your worries with them. Do what you did when you were young and imagine shapes and stories as they shift and change.

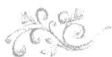

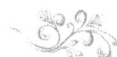

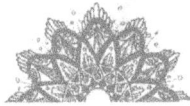

You have brains in your head. You have
feet in your shoes. You can steer
yourself any direction you choose.

– Dr Seuss

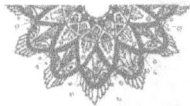

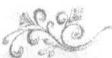 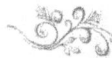

- Gaze at the stars. Look up at the beautiful night sky and appreciate the beauty of our wonderful galaxy.

- Learn a language. Evidence indicates that learning a new language can reduce your risk of dementia. Learning something new can help with mental health as well. Have a look at a short course near you, or consider an online workshop. Expand your horizons!

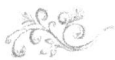

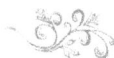

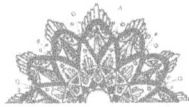

I was feeling crap and simply got a
blanket, put it on the grass of my front
lawn and lay down looking up into the
blue endless sky.
Worked like magic!

— Katrina

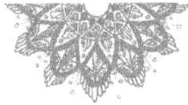

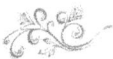 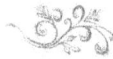

Digital detox. Switch off your computer and phone, daydream, be bored and allow your mind to wander.

Progressive muscle relaxation. Download an app or soundtrack to guide you through this calming and restorative process.

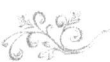

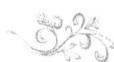

* _____

* _____

* _____

_____

_____

_____

Have you been outside today?

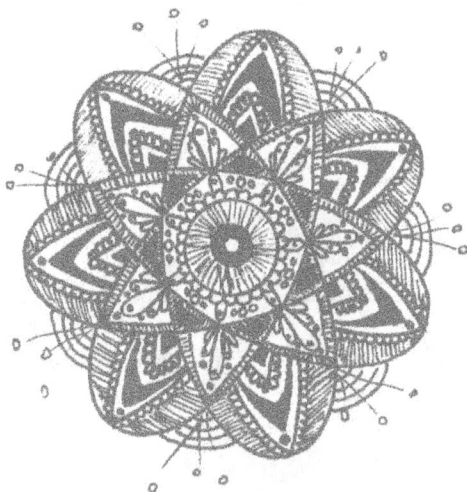

Chapter Three

Get Moving

*I*t may be the last thing you feel like doing, but you will be happy that you did.

Regular exercise has been shown to have very positive effects upon mental well-being. Whilst vigorous exercise releases endorphins (the "feel-good" chemicals that also alleviate pain) into our bloodstream, even gentle to moderate exercise increases serotonin, which has a number of benefits including lifting our mood and helping to counteract insomnia. The good news is that exercise doesn't need to be strenuous for us to feel some of its many benefits.

When you are stuck mentally, move physically. Here are some suggestions for getting moving.

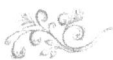 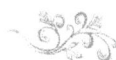

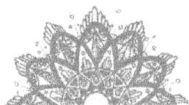

Those who think they have not time for
bodily exercise will sooner or later have
to find time for illness.

– Edward Stanley

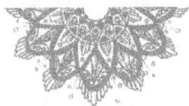

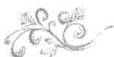 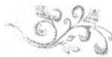

Walk. Even ten minutes will help. It's been scientifically proven that 30 minutes of walking is as effective as anti-depressants in treating mild to moderate depression. Just imagine how much better it will make you feel on a funk day! No one ever comes back from a walk and says, "I wish I didn't do that."

Dance. Jump, shake, jiggle and twist. Get your heart pumping, raise a sweat and lose yourself in the music. You could even dance naked for a full feeling of freedom. Sign up for a class of something new or revisit something you've loved before.

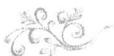

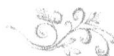

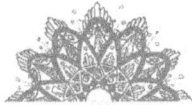

One of the happiest moments in life is
when you find the courage to let go of
what you can't change.

– Unknown

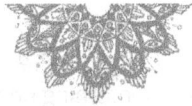

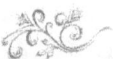
Have you been outside today?
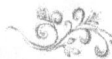

🌼 Yoga. If you aren't sure where to start and can't get to a class, there are plenty of videos available online that can get you going.

🌼 Tai chi. This is a gentle form of exercise combined with meditation.

🌼 Swim. Do laps, float, play and enjoy the weightlessness of your body in the water.

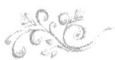

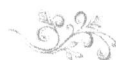

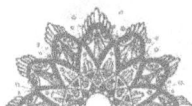

I've had the sort of day that would make
St. Francis of Assisi kick babies."

– Douglas Adams

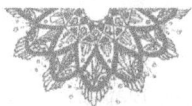

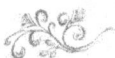

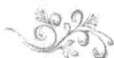

※ Go the beach. Get your toes in the sand, dip them in the ocean and take a gentle stroll. Afterwards sit and watch the waves flow in and out. The beach is great for restoring physical and mental balance.

※ Boxing. Whether you take it out on a punching bag or go to boxercise class, it's great therapy.

※ Bike. Get your bike out and go for a spin. Feel the breeze on your face and the wind in your hair, just like when you were a kid.

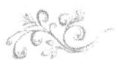

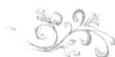

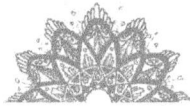

In three words I can sum up everything
I've learned about life. It goes on.

– Robert Frost

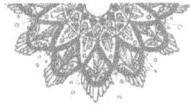

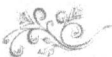 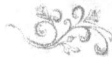

❀ Jump rope. Another fun childhood activity that's also a great cardio workout.

❀ Hula hoop. If you don't know how to do it, there are many great beginner videos online.

❀ Water aerobics. A great combination of dancing and being in the water.

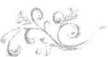

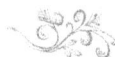

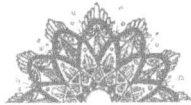

Prosperity makes friends, adversity
tries them.

– Publilius Syrus

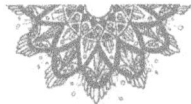

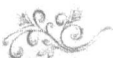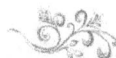

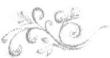 Water sports. Surfing, kayaking, skiing, paddle boarding – get moving, get wet and enjoy!

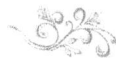 Fly a kite.

⁂ _____

⁂ _____

⁂ _____

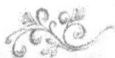 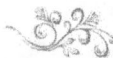

※ _____

※ _____

※ _____

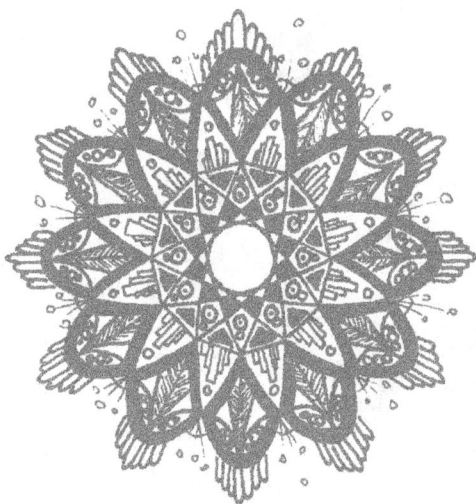

Chapter Four

Outside The House

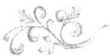 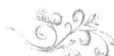

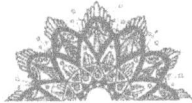

Courage doesn't always roar.
Sometimes courage is the quiet voice
at the end of the day, saying, "I will try
again tomorrow.".

– Mary Anne Radmacher

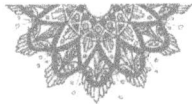

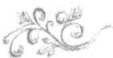

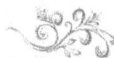

Get out of the house. It doesn't matter where. Go to the supermarket, shopping centre or just around the block. Just get out and give yourself a different view for a while.

Take yourself out for breakfast, lunch or dinner to a place you've always wanted to go. Dress up as if you're going on a date, because you are – with yourself. Enjoy every delicious mouthful.

People watch. Sit somewhere and observe the wonder of humanity walking and moving around you. Create stories in your mind of those who pass your way.

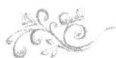

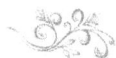

Have you been outside today?

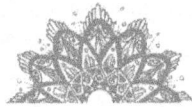

Outside the windows the day was bright: golden sunshine, blue sky, pleasant wind . . . I wanted to punch the happy day in the face, grab it by the hair, and beat it until it told me what the hell it was so happy about."

– Ilona Andrews

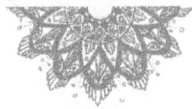

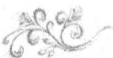

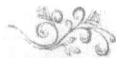

Find your closest waterfall. Lose yourself in the wonder of nature. An added bonus is that the environment close to a waterfall (and the ocean) has the perfect balance of negative ions, something we need more of in our electronics-filled environment.

Go to the movies. Find something you want to see and be sure to get yourself a big bucket of popcorn and an ice cream while you're at it.

Picnic. Pack up your lunch, grab a blanket and a book and find somewhere nice to sit, relax and enjoy.

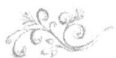

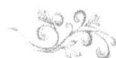

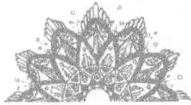

Nature is my go-to, be it a hike in the wilds, a swim or just sitting and watching the ocean. It helps ground me and get me out of a funk.

– Tasha

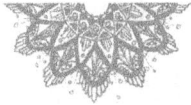

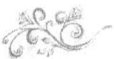 Have you been outside today?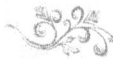

❋ Photography. Take photos of anything. Photography is a great mindfulness and gratitude practice.

❋ Go somewhere far from other people such as the beach or the bush. Yell, scream, cry – get it all out.

❋ Spend time surrounded by nature. There is growing evidence that access to the natural environment improves health and well-being, prevents disease and helps people recover from illness.

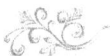 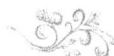

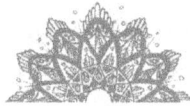

Calling my person. I have that one friend
with whom I can be brutally honest and
tell her exactly what I am feeling, no
matter how crazy it may sound. Knowing
that no judgement will be passed is
crucial for me and I assume for many
others..

– Elmina

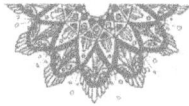

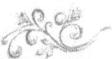 Have you been outside today?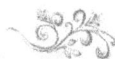

Take a walk in the forest or woods.

Visit a museum.

Visit an art gallery.

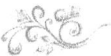

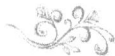

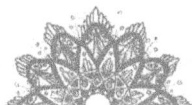

I am human and yeah I have very
bad days.

– Charlize Theron

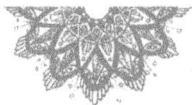

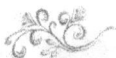

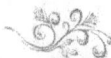

✤ Visit a relative.

✤ Do you have a favourite place/spot? If so, go there. If you don't have a regular spot, go somewhere that you have enjoyed visiting previously.

✤ Visit a nursing home as a volunteer. Take a resident for a stroll in the garden, read them a newspaper or just sit and listen.

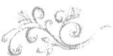

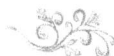

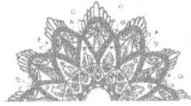

I remember asking the universe to crack me
open. I remember it like it was yesterday.
But it wasn't. It was lifetimes ago.

— Jacque

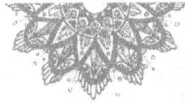

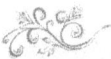 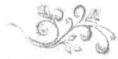

Fish. If you enjoy fishing, grab your rod and reel and throw a line or two.

Hang out with children. Kids can teach us so many things: mindfulness, being present, appreciation of the little things, acceptance of what is and – most importantly – how to have fun.

Go for a long drive – and get into some car karaoke! The louder the better. When stationary throw in some moves.

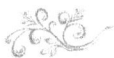

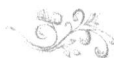

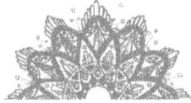

My go-to is definitely nature when a funk hits, and while not as often as it used to, it can still show up. I get grounded, I walk a lot, and eventually it passes. For me a big lesson has been in not getting emotionally attached to the funk. As I get older I realise the beauty in relativity, and that it takes the off days to have the on days, the lows to have the highs, and the hard work to reap the reward.

- Pru

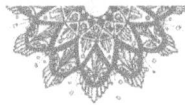

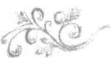
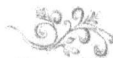

❋ _____

❋ _____

❋ _____

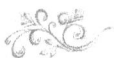

Have you been outside today?

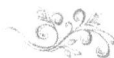

＊ _____

＊ _____

＊ _____

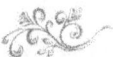 Have you been outside today?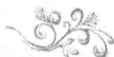

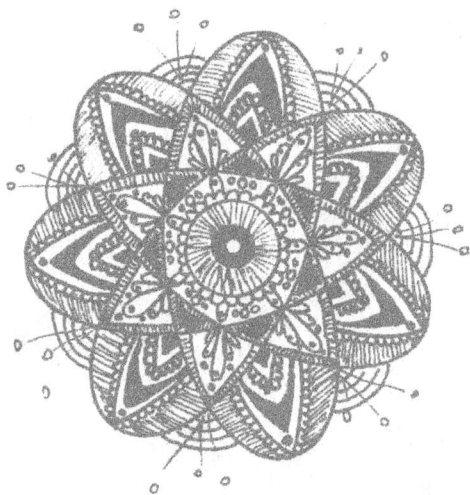

Chapter Five

Body Work

*S*ome people consider body treatments to be pampering. Try thinking of them as maintenance instead! Just like tuning up your car, body maintenance is required to keep us functioning and well-tuned.

These activities tend to get you out of your head and into your body and this can be a powerful mood booster. An added bonus is they tend to feel great too!

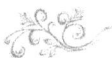 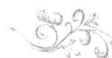

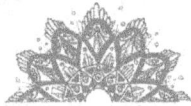

Do something every day that is loving
toward your body and gives you the
opportunity to enjoy the sensations of
your body

– Golda Poretsky

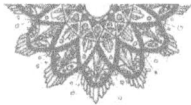

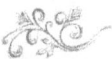 Have you been outside today?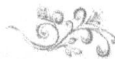

Massage. There's nothing quite like a massage to bring you back into your body. It will leave you feeling floaty and blissful and you'll sleep better afterwards.

Reflexology. A system of massage used to relieve tension and treat illness, based on the theory that there are reflex points on the feet, hands, and head linked to every part of the body. A foot rub of any kind always feels amazing.

Acupuncture. A part of traditional Chinese medicine, acupuncture consists of inserting fine needles into specific points on the skin. Performed by a skilled practitioner, acupuncture can be a safe and effective treatment for a range of disorders.

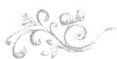

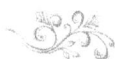

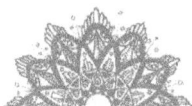

We have nothing to be ashamed of. We are actually warriors, and only we know the strength it takes to ask for help, pull ourselves out of our funks and continue living and smiling and being in the world.

– Aylee

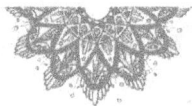

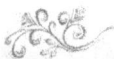 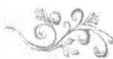

Reiki. A Japanese technique for stress reduction and relaxation that also promotes healing.

Bowen therapy. A holistic remedial body technique that works on the soft connective tissue (fascia) of the body. Bowen therapy can be used to treat musculoskeletal or related neurological problems, including acute sports injuries and chronic or organic conditions.

Float tank. This is essentially a way of achieving deep relaxation by spending an hour or more lying quietly in darkness, suspended in a solution of warm water and Epsom salts.

Indulge in some body pampering such as a facial, body scrub, pedicure or manicure. It's a wonderful way to relax, feel special and take time out for yourself.

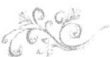

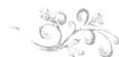

Have you been outside today?

———————————————————————————————

———————————————————————————————

———————————————————————————————

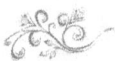 Have you been outside today?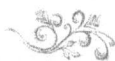

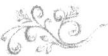
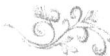
Have you been outside today?

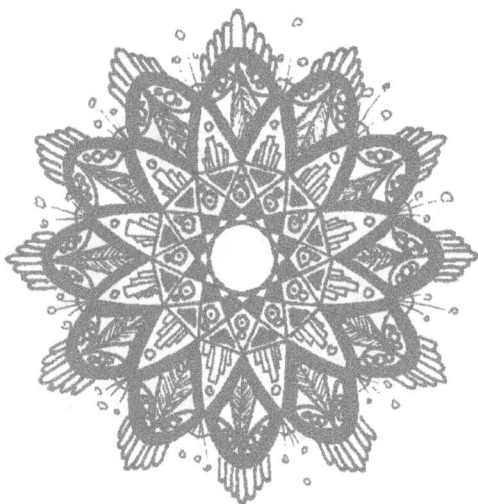

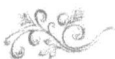

Have you been outside today?

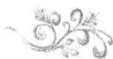

Chapter Six

Keeping The Funky Days At Bay

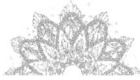

How we care for ourselves gives our brain
messages that shape our self-worth so we
must care for ourselves in every way, every day.

Sam Owen

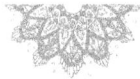

W hether or not you have been diagnosed with a mental illness, one thing to remember is that funky days will come and go. They may not stick around for long, but they are an occasional part of life, and when they are over, life is so much brighter for it.

The good news is that there are some things you can do to help keep them at bay.

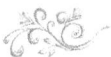 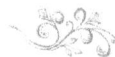

Here are 12 strategies that I have found useful for maintaining good mental health. The nice thing about them is that they usually feel good when you are doing them, and the effects linger afterwards as well.

- Sleep – getting adequate good quality sleep is one of the most important things you can do to maintain good physical and mental health. There is no right amount; everybody is different. Find out what works for you and do your best to get that every night.

- Move – move your body for 30 minutes a day. Find something you enjoy and do that. It doesn't have to cost money: walk, dance, stretch – just move.

- Nourish – eat the healthiest food you can afford, preferably as close to nature as possible.

- Hydrate – drink good clean drinking water, or refreshing herbal teas. Drink whatever nourishes you.

- Breathe – get outside into nature as much as possible. Mother nature is a wonderful healer.

- Meditation – start with just three minutes a day. It doesn't have to be complicated; just notice the breath moving in and out of your nostrils.

- Give thanks – notice and give thanks for what makes you grateful.

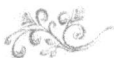

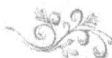

- Be kind – do random acts of kindness whenever you can.

- Give – doing volunteer work on a regular basis can help take the focus off you. The giver usually benefits more than the receiver.

- Time out – book yourself a regular mental health day, and on that day do whatever your heart desires.

- Educate – maintain the curiosity of a child and never stop learning. Attend courses, try new things, extend yourself, step out of your comfort zone and choose a topic you've never considered before. As Ghandi so wisely said: "Live as if you were to die tomorrow; learn as if you were to live forever."

- Write – keep a journal, start a blog, write in a diary. Getting your thoughts on paper is cathartic and healing.

If you have been feeling low in mood for two weeks or more, it's a good idea to see your GP for a check-up.

There are many things that can contribute to a persistent low mood and the sooner you get them checked out and seen to, the quicker you'll feel better.

Although this book was written for everyone, if you have been diagnosed with depression and/or anxiety, there

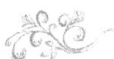 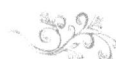

are many organisations that have helpful free resources available online.

Please visit my website at www.transpiral.com.au for a current list of links to places I find useful.

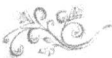

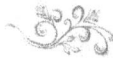

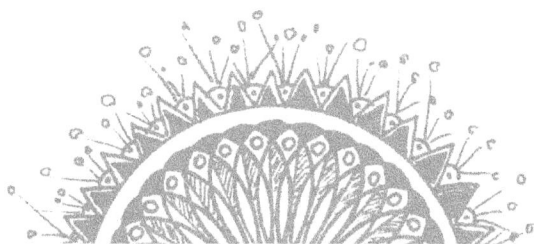

Personal Stories

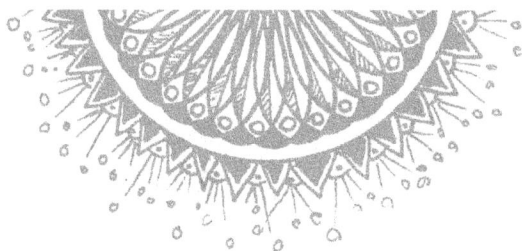

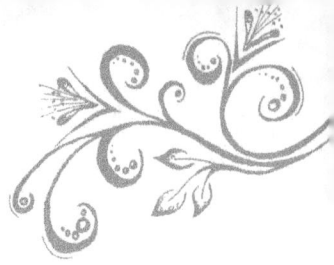

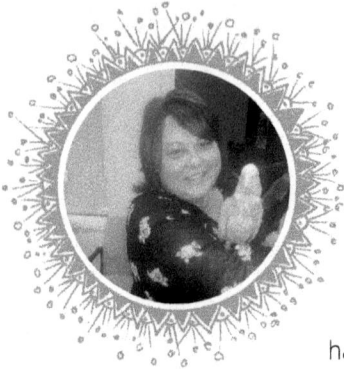

Angela

I've personally been visited by the black dog recently. I am still working hard on sending him to the pound as I've had enough pet therapy from him in the last year!

There are a couple of things I've learned. Firstly, don't be ashamed to take meds. Secondly, don't feel guilty for the way you feel. It's not your fault. It's important to put yourself first and don't take unrealistic advice from people who really have no idea how it feels.

The very best thing for me was to eat healthy. I asked my husband to take a month off work to care for me and manage the kids and the house. It's given me time to put good food (prepared by my husband) into my body. I'm taking baby steps and resting when I'm tired, without any guilt or responsibility. It's been like being in my very own health farm and mental institution without having my door locked at 7pm and forced to do craft with sedated people.

I'm still on the journey. I'm slowly doing things again. I feel proud if I just do a basic chore in the house, like cook a meal for the family.

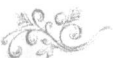

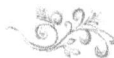

Have you been outside today?

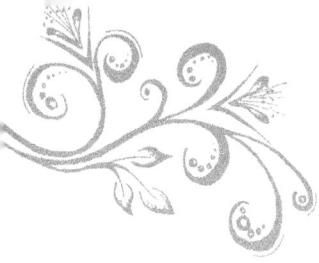

Laura

I wanted to share something beautiful my mum did for me when I was in a funk. I had an awful experience about seven years ago when living in remote Western Australia. It was so awful; I struggled to talk about it and struggled to be around close friends (the more I tried to communicate my feelings the more I realised how alone I was because nobody understood). I was so down, all I could do was submerse myself in new environments to distract me from my distress.

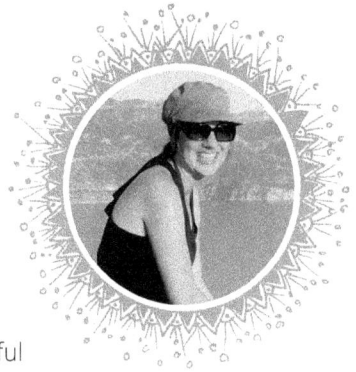

My mum made me a key chain with specially chosen positive affirmations to carry with me wherever I went. She typed them, printed them on different coloured card, laminated them and put them on a key chain. It was probably the most amazing gift I've ever received. I carried it wherever I went and read them over and over again, especially when I tore myself up and consumed myself with the past.

Every time my mind wanted to believe the other side of the story – that there was a massive bully destroying me – those affirmations reminded me of the person I am, the love I have in my life and helped to keep me grounded.

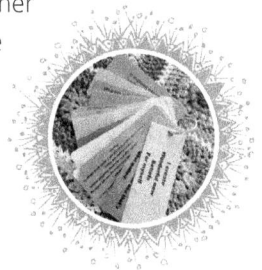

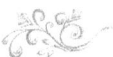

Have you been outside today?

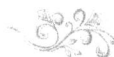

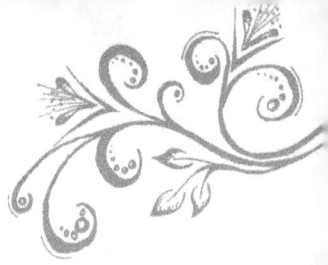

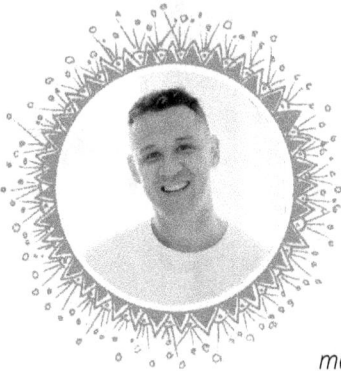

Jamie

www.scanphilosophy.com

My goodness! There have been *many* funk days in my life! Although one thing I always try and remember when I am having one is that I have actually had less funk days than awesome days. But sometimes we dwell in the dark rather than shining in the light – so that is one thing that gets me through.

I have always held a firm belief that a lot of the story we are here to tell is already written. Some chapters are blank; some are a "choose your own adventure". But it is all travelling from point A to point B – the beginning and the end are the same for all of us. Birth, then death. I believe that everything that happens to us in life is a part of something much bigger and our job is to be still and feel what that is and go in that direction. It is also our job to pay attention to when we are feeling restless, not ourselves, just a bit off, because that is our higher calling telling us we need to make a change, be it large or small.

Knowing that everything is going to be OK is also something that I keep in the forefront of my mind. We've all faced some less than desirable situations in life, and ultimately, we got through it because we are here today telling our stories, or reading others' stories. So we must always hold on to that

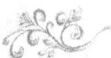 Have you been outside today?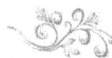

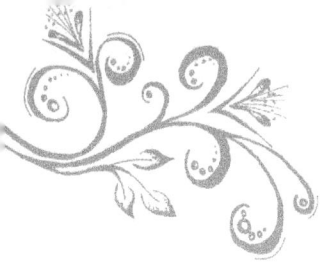

knowing that it is all going to be OK in the end. Sometimes we are not always where we want to be in life, but we are always where we are meant to be; it's just a matter of going deep inside ourselves and figuring out what that is. What is the lesson? What are the opportunities in this moment to go in a different direction?

These are some of my handy hints that get me through the funk days!

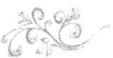

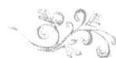

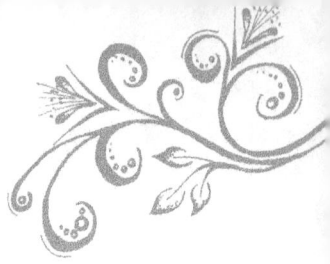

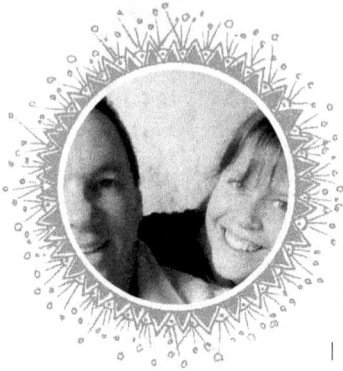

Erica

As one who travels with anxiety, and skirts the rim of depression, I would love to share one or two survival tips.

Depression is an unwanted visitor who arrives without notice and outstays her welcome. Anxiety I have always lived with. I have learnt how to navigate my way through a world full of obstacles. I stay away from crowds when I am tired. I try not to shop when anxious, or I end up with a trolley full of *stuff* that I have no idea what it is or what it is for. I then have to return it and get a refund. I no longer even bother making up stories, I just say that I changed my mind.

If everything gets too busy, I stop. I slow it down. I take one small step at a time. If that is all that I can handle, then that is all that I can handle. Keep breaking it down into steps or stages that do not overwhelm me. That is how I have learnt to navigate anxiety.

Depression is black hole that can take years to emerge from. When I was deep in the hole, I did not know if I would survive. It was dark. It was scary. There were no sides. There was no light. I could not think. I could not feel. I could not do anything. I could not be anything. I was gone.

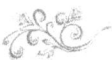

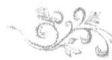

Have you been outside today?

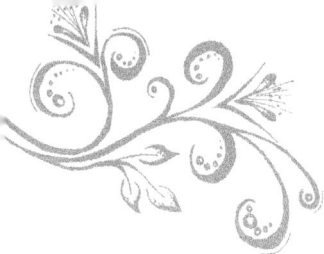

Depression crushed me when my body would not or could not conceive a child. My heart broke and my mind broke at my body's betrayal. I had babysat since the age of 12 and I had always imagined a home full of harum-scarum boys who would tumble over themselves to receive Mum's hug.

The children never came.

We were living remote and travelling to Alice Springs for rounds of Chlomid. My hormones and emotions raged. My husband didn't know how to handle the mood swings. He did not know how to be there for me. I was away from my mum and all that was familiar. I loved where we lived but was more alone than ever.

My husband is a survivor – an adult survivor of child abuse. Even his being here on this planet is a miracle. He is not a suicide statistic or an alcoholic or a drug addict. But he is not or was not emotionally equipped to deal with what I was going through. I remember a still quiet voice, calm in the maelstrom of depression, stating that I would have to get myself through this.

That was the hard part, going through. There is no hiding, no skirting the issues, no side-tracking. I had to face myself and work through the long hard emotions.

As the hormones raged and tried to make my body ovulate to conceive a much wanted red-haired child, I could have

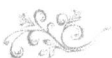

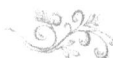

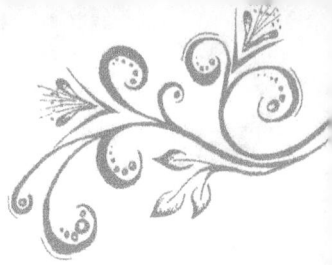

walked into the desert, especially on a star-strewn night, and never returned.

There were days when emerging from bed was an achievement in itself. Having a busy astronomy business to run and star talks to deliver meant I had to function. Having a husband who loved me but did not know what to do to be there for me nearly destroyed us. I would rage at my husband, Timbo; at myself; at the sky. I did not know the way forward.

I did not have access to resources. I worked out that the insufficient help from a different mental health nurse every month at Yulara was not going to work. I did not know what would help.

The RSPCA's website, with their dogs of the month, was my salvation. Choosing Redley, an 18-month-old red heeler-cairn terrier cross, allowed me to pour my love into an intelligent, sentient being who needed me and my love. I had to get up. I had to walk Redley. We both adjusted to each other. We were both anxious; both needed to love and be loved.

My teddy bear with long legs never left my side. Redley sat on his own office chair as I worked on rosters and paperwork. He rode in the ute with me as I delivered telescopes to the sites around the resort. He walked the sand dunes with me, snuffling and exploring. Tracking lizards, chasing corellas, becoming confident with his jaunty strut and his feathered

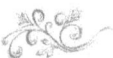

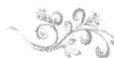

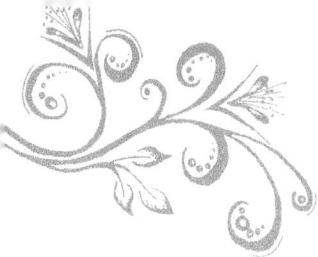

tail held high. Redley was and is my fur kid, not a substitute, but a much loved member of my family.

Having someone to love, and keeping active, are what Redley gave me. Instead of being painted into a corner, where the black paint eliminates the white tiles and the red exit signs, Redley lit the way forward. I did not need to see the whole road. I just needed to see the next few steps.

Learning how to find joy in small things opened cracks and allowed slivers of happiness in. Walking at dawn, exploring the beauty of sunrise and early bird tracks, snake slitherings, and lizard dances across the cool red sand. Instead of being immune to the praise that came after a fabulous star talk, I could say, "Thank you."

Saying thank you for small steps is the way that I have kept going. When I think I have nothing to appreciate, I give thanks that my feet work, that my ankles work, that my knees might be a bit dodgy but they still get me up the hill. I give thanks for every part of my body that allows me to function and I give thanks to the Creator of all things for allowing me to be a part of creation.

The children never came, however there are different ways to have children in my life. Tim and I are honorary aunt and uncle to our friends' children. Our own nieces and nephews have grown. I plan to be a Pyjama Angel, a tutor to a child in foster care, once the latest health issues are sorted.

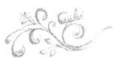

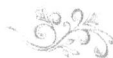

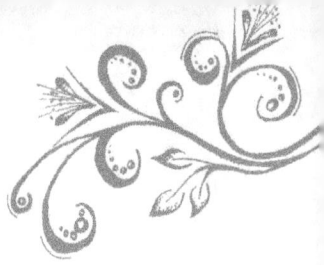

Ten years on, Redley, Tim and I have weathered illnesses and numerous moves. Tim and I have survived due to the fact that we were and always are friends first. He is my darling Timbo and he knows now how to be there for me. Redley is over 12 years old. A bit stiff in the legs and a tad night blind; however he is still delightfully fluffy and still brings joy to my days.

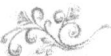

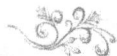

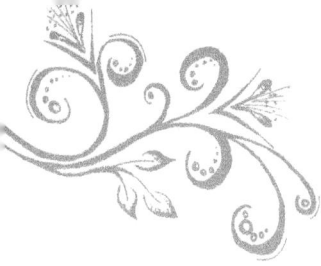

Meekehleh Connors Deserio

Author, writer, mentor, healer

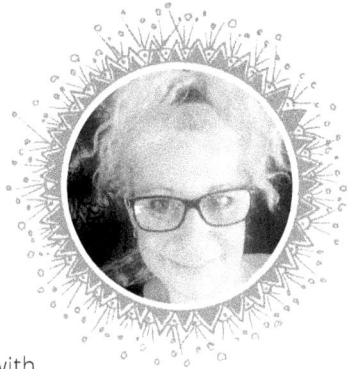

As someone who has suffered with depression and anxiety for most of my life, I have tried many different methods to boost my mood, and heal my mind; or at the very least find coping mechanisms that work for me.

I'm a writer, so my go-to plan is always to write or create something arty. From journaling how I'm feeling, to writing a blog post or working on one of the four different books I am writing simultaneously, I make sure I immerse myself in something good. I nourish my soul. It's not always about writing down how I'm feeling; sometimes the best thing is to distance myself from it altogether. Getting busy means that when I look up, I realise that several hours have passed, maybe even only half an hour, and I feel better.

My motto is: *Bite off more than you can chew, and then chew like mad!* I've always been this way. I find that a mind that has too much time to think tends to start spinning. It's better to be busy and active! Busyness quells that anxious mind from working overtime and sending me spiralling into an uncontrollable pit of despair. And so I study. I have already obtained seven diplomas and certificates, and now, at the age of 47, I am working towards a double degree in law/arts,

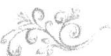

Have you been outside today?

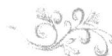

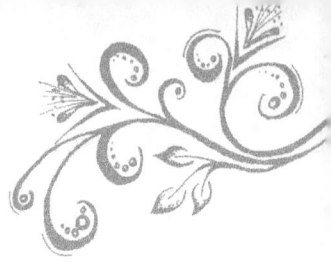

which will take me approximately five years to complete. I finally feel like I am doing what I was always supposed to be doing, and that does my mental health a world of good.

Goal setting and working towards something where I can dangle the carrot (such as planning a holiday or mini retreat) always works really well in inspiring feelings of well-being; even just a night away in a hotel room – just me, my favourite snacks and the chance to write, read, dream, plan and reconnect. This works wonders when I need it most, especially when I can breathe out with a view of the beach, the mountains or the city skyline. That is bliss to me.

The seaside has always been my place to unwind. Having grown up by the water, it's the one corner of this busy world where I find peace and equilibrium once again. It renews, refreshes, rejuvenates and restores, and spurs me on to better things. But I also find joy in other places that truly mean something to me: sitting staring at the glittering Manhattan skyline ignites my soul, as do Brokenback mountain range in New South Wales' Hunter Valley and the beaches of Vanuatu – but all for different reasons. Often there is nothing better than immersing yourself in the electric vibe of the city. At other times, the only antidote for the tough times is to get back to nature, feel the grass, breathe in the fresh air, sit in the sun, and let all of the negativity melt away with the warmth of the day.

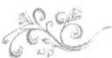

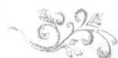

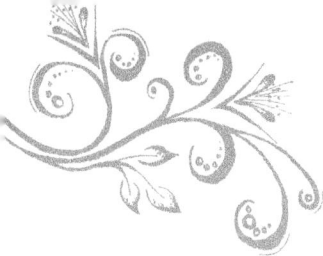

I read. I play music (driving to a new destination to take photos, and playing it really loud!). At home, I meditate. I light candles. I make the room fragrant with lavender. I exercise it out (I joined the gym). I sit with the magic of crystals. I pray. I seek out the people in my tribe who inspire me on to better things and soothe my soul. I do courses in healing. And I have created a bedroom (the spot where I do most of my work) that is full of vibrant colours, keepsakes, and pretty things that invite creativity. My bedroom exudes an atmosphere of love and homeliness, a sense of belonging and peace. It is my haven from the world.

And when I must – I disconnect. I switch off my phone. I disengage from the internet, and especially social media, far away from the distractions and bad news of the world. I grab a blanket that I chose specifically for warmth and comfort, I make a hot chocolate and I put on a movie and I forget about life for a while.

Making new memories, taking my kids places and tasting as much of life as I possibly can – enriching experiences that become something to write about and share and focus on in positive ways – is how I've lived my life for many years. Travelling, expanding my heart and mind, working towards helping others who are less fortunate than me, sending love out into the world: these are a real blessing and have been part and parcel of how I have managed to navigate some very dark and difficult times in my life.

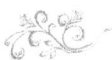

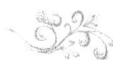

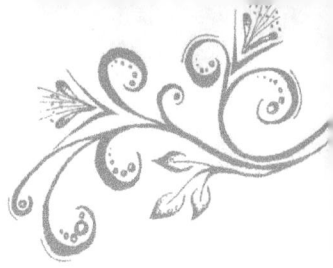

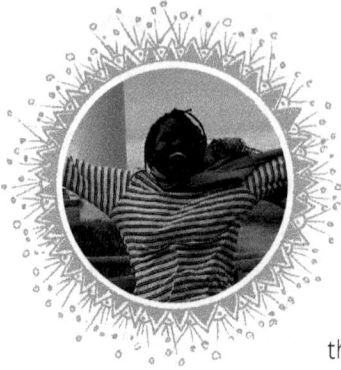

Noma

Noddy and Winnie the Pooh – these characters have more times than not got me out of a funk. I reach for these books and things don't seem quite as bad. I was in a bad way after a hysterectomy procedure and my friend Wendy visited with nuts and Winnie the Pooh in tow. Since then, whenever I am out of sync I reach for those favourite children's storybooks. Sometimes I like to visit the library - teenage fiction section does the trick. My latest read that got me out of the gloom is *It's OK, I'm wearing really big knickers!* by Louise Rennison.

My discovery of how books can help me comes after 30 years of psychologists and anti-depressants.

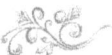 Have you been outside today?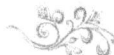

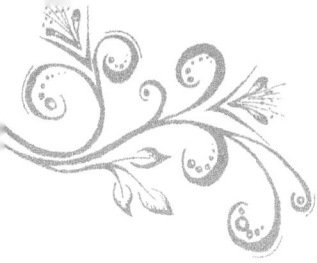

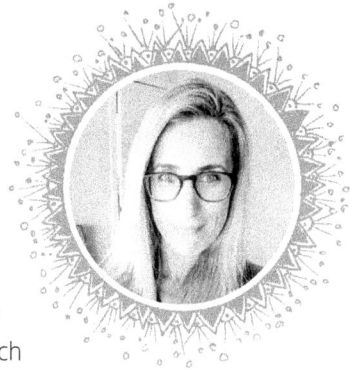

Elmina

Recently I was in a funk – a funk of all sorts. A funk which came on quite abruptly and very much uninvited – ha. Are they ever invited?!

I felt like the world was closing in on me; I was overwhelmed by my own skin. I felt that tightness in the chest, the racing mind, the relentless worry about everything and anything. My funk was brought on by one particular event. Usually I would just carry on, and not even give it any time – but this time around all I did was give it time.

The funk was brought on because I didn't move to the countryside. This was my grand plan – it was to be my year ahead. Life plan sorted. TICK. My way out of the very claustrophobic city, the busyness which seemed to consume my space. When this fell through I was in all sorts of funk. This was my escape! What now? Stay here? Move out on my own? Go overseas – which is always the fall-back plan – my escape plan in life, move overseas. So began my around three months of super funk, not wanting to go to work, nothing was enough.

There was something missing in everything. I was not loving my job, my home and the place I lived in. My usual supports weren't around me. My family back home did what they

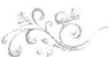

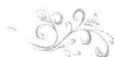

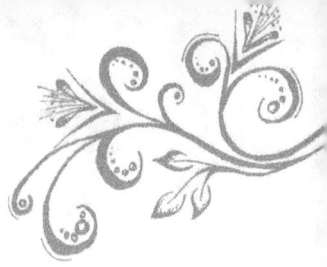

could, and encouraged me about work, but I wasn't fully honest with them how hard this hit me. I was lost.

To find my way back to me: so began my journey, which I carry on today. I set off to a boot camp for the mind, a short three-day meditation retreat which re-fired my practice. I sought out advice from friends, in particular people current in my life, the housemate, the bestie, the new friend, the old friend. I was in search of answers from all perspectives to see if I could put the jigsaw pieces together – to move forward. To move on. To calm the mind and get rid of this never-ending anxiety.

I started meditating every day for 30 minutes, collected all the intel on myself I could, and yes, things were said to me which were new, old and jarring, but I needed to hear it. I worked out that I was so focused on what didn't happen that I wasn't tuning in to what *was* happening. After a short holiday where my yoga practice was re-inspired, I came back with confidence – and I hadn't even realised that I had lost my confidence.

Gratefulness came back. I was grateful for all the things that I had, and I put to sleep the anxiety of all the things I didn't have. Passion for the work I do came back; compassion for the people we serve was re-inspired. Being thankful for the home I do live in, the wonderful human being I get to share it with and the wonderful human beings who I share my life

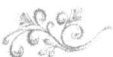

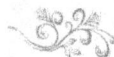

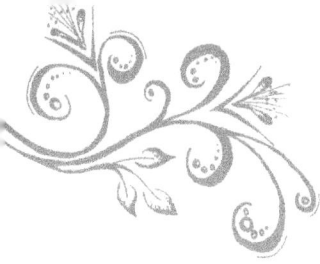

with. I am content. I got the mind space I needed and I am more comfortable with being kind to me.

These are the things I do to get myself out of a funk.

- Music. Listening to music and then dancing, just letting go and dancing in the living room, in the bedroom, in the office early in the morning when no one is in! I dance like no-one's watching me and if someone catches me well that's that! Recently I sent a video of me free dancing in the living room to a friend – I shared with her my crazy dance!

- Reading Brené Brown – re-visiting my favourite chapters in her books. When I'm in a huge funk I read the whole book. I remind myself that I am not the only one suffering today; there are others.

- Hitting the gym for a run or cycle class. These days this has been replaced by yoga and meditation – but for many years the gym and vigorous exercise was brilliant.

- Slowing myself down and seeing why I am in a funk. I can only do this if I'm in the right state of mind though, because let's face it, breaking it down for yourself when in a funk can just lead to a whole lot more funk!

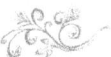

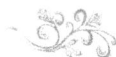

Have you been outside today?

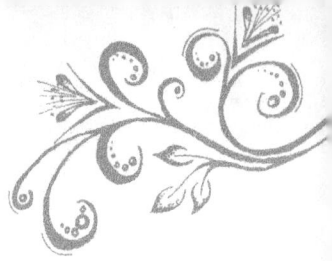

❋ Calling my person. I have that one friend with whom I can be brutally honest and tell her exactly what I am feeling, no matter how crazy it may sound. Knowing that no judgement will be passed is crucial for me and I assume for many others. I don't have many people that I think do well when I am in a funk, but those that are there – a couple of them are truly amazing.

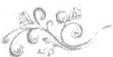

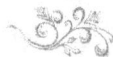

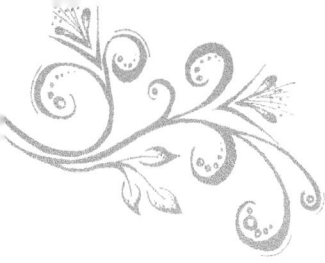

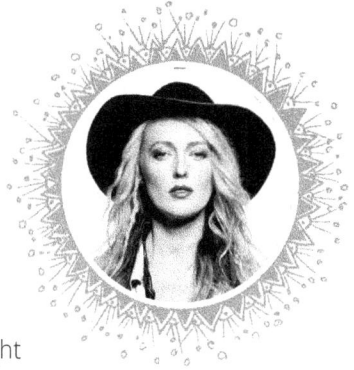

Bron

My boyfriend of three-and-a-half years died in a motorbike accident aged 24. When I thought life had turned for the better, I married an abusive drug addict, launching into marriage after only knowing him for six weeks (when he proposed). Made millions of dollars, then lost it all and started again. Hit rock bottom entirely after working my ring off throughout my 20s. Worked day and night to build up an empire that ultimately didn't end up in my hands. Wanted to end it all. If it wasn't for family and a few close mates I would've ended it – for sure. Depression and alcoholism run in my family. I have never been diagnosed and think any bouts of depression have been more situational. There were definitely a few key things that helped me then and still help me now if I have an off day.

The things that helped me:

❀ Finally focusing on my own dreams and not someone else's.

❀ Travelling and saying yes to every opportunity I could.

❀ Writing down everything I want to do before I die, and implementing them.

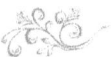

Have you been outside today?

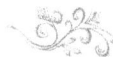

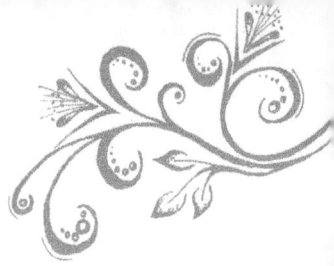

- Having a "universe board" (visible goals) that I see every single day when I wake up.

- Jumping in the ocean, even when it's cold!

- Fucking off negative energy, people that drain you, use you or don't keep their commitments.

- Becoming a leader, so you have people that look up to you. It makes you want to be a better person.

- Being honest with myself and others.

- Having long periods where I don't drink alcohol also helped.

- I have things I do every day, but not enough. Silly things, like thinking about what I appreciate about my life, myself etc.

- Making time to do nothing without feeling guilty (I still struggle with this) – like sitting in the sun!

- Call a friend.

- Write a song.

My life is completely different now. I live in Byron Bay , run my own company, play (and now release) music, have an incredibly loving and supportive partner, am healthy and have the best friends in the world. Life couldn't be better

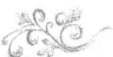

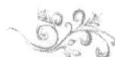

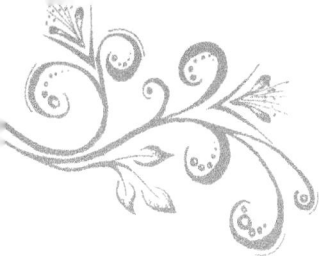

really, but even in all its imperfect perfection, I still have my off days. I think when you have reached the depths of the darkness, it is easy to go back there. Of course, emotionally "safe" people don't allow, or acknowledge, they have dark days, but like an anti-depressant (I'm speculating here as I have never had one) it numbs out both the good and the bad if you don't acknowledge feelings. I think it is a blessing to feel deeply. We must make sure we leave room for joy too.

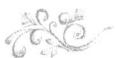

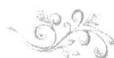

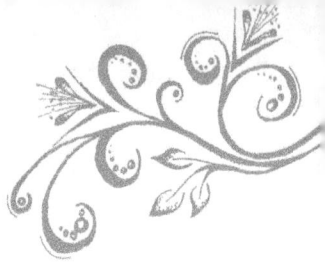

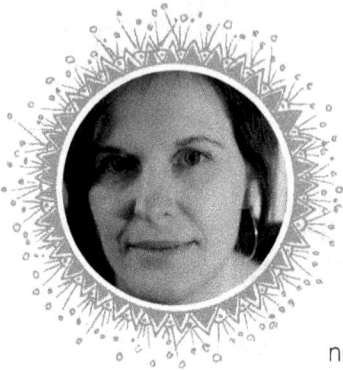

Waratah

I realised recently that so much of my lifestyle habits are born from a need to quieten a really active mind. Someone said to me recently that they couldn't control their light and darkness; I don't think any of us have mastered that. There are, however, coping strategies that are healthy and life-affirming that will eventually lead us out of darkness. And there are those that will continue to lead us down the rabbit hole to shame, guilt and self-denigration.

For the most part, I choose ones that will help me quieten my mind which usually involves movement – walking up a mountain or dancing are two of my favourites when life gets really noisy inside. When I am not in full freak-out mode I turn to yoga and meditation.

One of the things I have noticed in both myself and my clients and students is that when we 'need' our practice the most is quite often when we abandon it. I have made it a point to know when the freak-out is escalating and take action. Even going for a walk around the block can help to gain a new perspective.

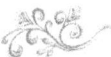

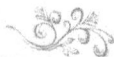

Have you been outside today?

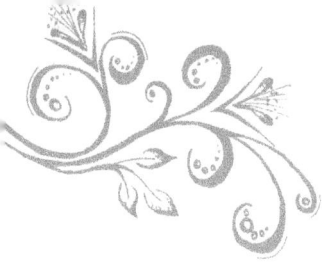

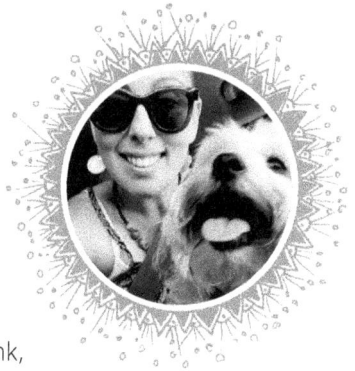

Aylee

My best friend Rae-Anne asked me to write about the things that help me most when I'm in a funk, or in my case, what helps me when I'm depressed. Funks are a normal part of life; depression is a funk that you can't shake. You may send it on its way for a moment but it's always there.

It's just the way I was created I think; a sensitive soul with a lot of responsibility and stress placed upon me from an early age, exacerbated by genetic predisposition and a lot of struggles. You see, I have suffered from depression from about the age of ten and continue to struggle with it most days. I live with chronic pain and illness so that adds to my feelings of low self-worth, frustration, despair and sometimes total defeat – so much so that I have been suicidal. When you live this way you learn ways to motivate yourself to continue with your life.

It sounds extreme but it's true. I once read a quote that said, "The bravest thing I ever did was continuing my life when I wanted to die." Without a list of things to do to overcome my bad days I wouldn't be here. Some of my coping mechanisms are positive and some are just that – "coping mechanisms" – and some may say that they do more harm than good (insert coffee and cake here!) but when you struggle with pain, depression and fatigue it's a pretty tortuous combination.

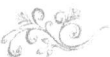

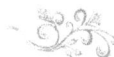

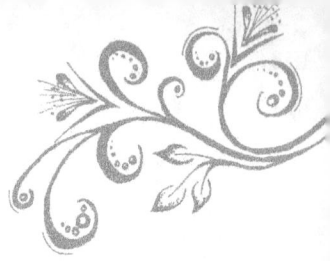

So I do the best I can with what I have, what I know and what I can manage.

Speaking of coffee and cake here is my list, and in no order of preference. OK, coffee and cake is first!

- Get out of the house and go and sit in a café and have coffee and cake. This helps me to feel connected to the world and as I watch people going about their business and see people connecting and talking I feel less alone. And yes, of course the yummy coffee and cake helps release some feel-good chemicals!

- Sleep – I do a lot of this even when I don't want to, so I have a bit of a love-hate relationship with sleep. But when days are really bad sleep can be my only respite.

- Music, music and more music – I love listening to positive music and singing loudly either in my car or at home. If I can dance at the same time it's even better! Dancing is actually my biggest love and the fact that I cannot do it much anymore bears a heavy weight on my happiness. So sometimes I just push through the pain and shake my groove thang – and I always feel amazing at the time. The aftermath isn't pleasant but still worth it most of the time.

- Walk – usually with dogs as they make me happy. Even when the pain is bad walking is so bloody good, and if you

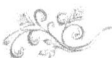

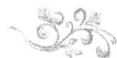

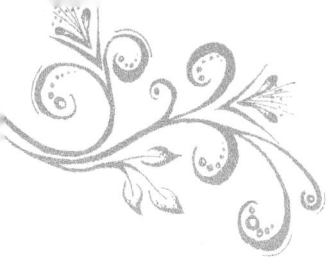

walk without too much suffering don't ever take your legs for granted – please! I miss this terribly.

- Doggies – I am very blessed to look after other people's doggies and they make me so happy, I mean *really* happy. My husband says I don't ever laugh like I do when I'm with my doggies. Their kisses, cuddles, wet noses and wagging tails fill my heart with love and just looking at them and patting them brings me peace.

- Sunshine – and if you combine that with coffee and cake, dogs and music, it's even more glorious!

- Talk to my husband and tell him I'm feeling down and just cry while he holds me. He always makes me feel better.

- Cry – this is so important! I always feel better after I've cried and in fact I'm writing this list after having done a few of these things. I called my husband and had a good cry, then had a really long shower, now I'm sitting outside in the sunshine writing. Oooh, that reminds me of another thing...

- Writing – I don't do it often enough which is crazy because it helps immensely. I love writing without care for grammar or spelling (so I stay in the flow) and I just let the feelings roll out. I often start with the angry feelings and then manage to find myself calmer as I keep writing.

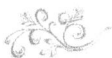

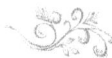

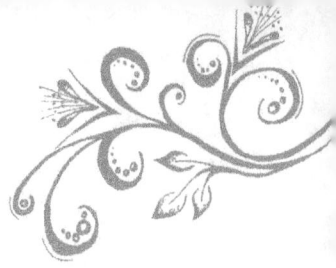

- Talking to Spirit – I do this through writing mostly and sometimes whilst lying down either in bed, or in a nice spot in nature (I did it a few weeks ago in the park and it was very powerful). I ask Spirit questions and the answers come so clear and I feel so much calmer and centered and peaceful and motivated and so many other things. It may sound crazy to some but I know that this is where I get my most incredible insights and validations and ideas and reassurance – but sadly I don't do this as often as I should. (Note to self: "DO THIS MORE OFTEN!")

- Talk to friends – I only do this with a few people and Rae-Anne is one of them.

- Shower – loooooong hot showers ... ahhh!

- Gratitude – reminding myself of all the things I have to be grateful for in my life. This could be a list or sometimes it's just looking at my husband and thinking, *Wow, I'm so grateful to have him in my life*, or looking at the flowers in my garden. Watching my garden grow and bloom brings me a lot of joy. Even if I need to delegate the actual gardening duties to my hubby, I am the one that appreciates the end result.

- The beach – nothing clears the soul like an ocean swim (followed by an iced coffee!).

- Movies – Netflix and I are in a relationship!

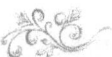 Have you been outside today?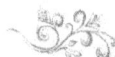

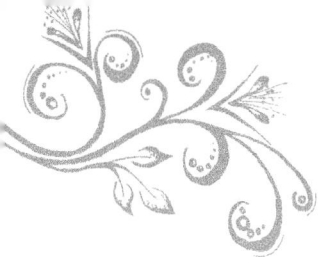

- Watch videos of my niece – my two-year-old niece is the light of my life. As we don't live in the same state I don't get to see her as much as I would like so the videos her parents send me are my most favourite gift. I watch them over and over and they bring me right out my funk and into pure joy in an instant. When everything seems helpless and I can't see the light I just think of her and my life has meaning, purpose and joy again. Being an aunty is my favourite thing in the whole wide world!

- Help others – it sounds cliché but for me it means everything. Helping others reminds me of why I am here on this earth and that I have much to share and that my struggles haven't been for nothing; they have given me great insight, awareness and strength and compassion for other human beings.

If I were sitting in a café right now writing this list nobody would ever know that an hour ago I was lying on the floor crying and feeling like my life had no meaning or purpose or joy or anything for that matter. I was numb and panicking and wanted to escape my reality. This is the roller coaster of my life, and the lives of many of us who have depression or ongoing funky days.

We have nothing to be ashamed of. We are actually warriors! Only we know the strength it takes to ask for help, pull ourselves out of our funks and continue living, smiling and

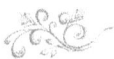

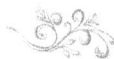

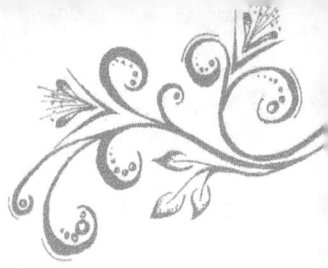

being in the world and trying to contribute to it in some way. Whether through work or family, as a husband or wife or even as a friend. We need to be proud of ourselves and of each other for showing up even when we don't want to.

May this book show us that we are never alone and that there are always things we can do to shift our focus.

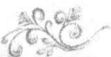

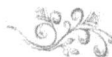

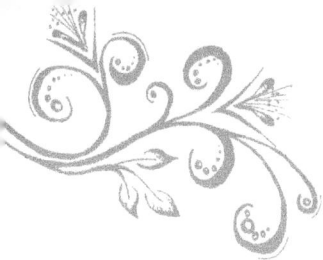

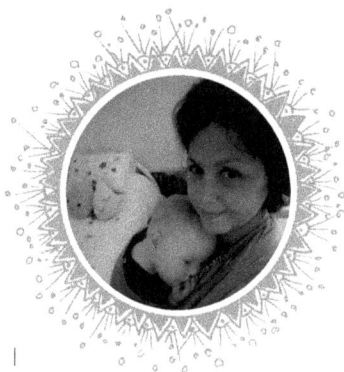

Leah

I think I will always be aware of my
predisposition towards depression,
and there are certain situations I
actively avoid to protect myself. First of all,
let me back up and give a bit of context.

I am an adoptee, with all the textbook neuroses and
insecurities that they write about children of adoption. I
was raised in a middle-class family, went to private schools,
and shared my family's discomfort with dysfunction and
"complicated" lives. I married young and had three attractive,
smart children. I was probably a bit of a smug shit, truth be
known, even if I kept my sense of superiority to myself.

My second child, my first son, was a smart and precocious
child. Easy at home, but frequently in trouble at school. I
remember the uneasy feeling I had when his Year 3 teacher
reported that he had said "it was like there were voices in
his head telling him to do the wrong thing". Maybe it was
nothing, but I remember the sense of dread I felt hearing it.

Fast forward to my son at age 17, heartbroken over his first
love lost, and dabbling in marijuana with school mates. It's
always hard to know as a parent what is normal difficult
teenage behaviour and what starts to signal an actual
problem, but Ben became gradually more paranoid and

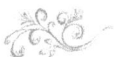

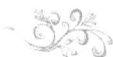

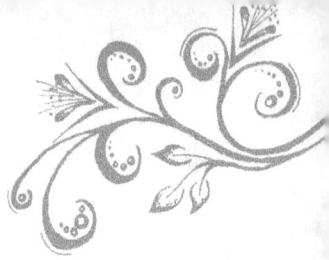

angry. He eventually had a major psychotic episode and was hospitalised. What followed was three years of constant admissions, stints of homelessness when he was not safe to have in our home, and an eventual diagnosis of schizophrenia.

I tell his story because it is interwoven with my own. I found, to my dismay, that I was completely ill-equipped, both personally and socially, to travel this road. As difficult as dealing with his illness was – along with the fighting with mental health teams for support, the meetings with doctors and social workers, care plan meetings that went nowhere – it was manageable. What I couldn't manage was the shame that this was happening to me. This stuff happened to other people. To uneducated people with no resources. Not to me with my clever beautiful children who allowed me to dutifully drag them to church every week.

I had become the person I'd casually blown off in the past, and now my friends did the same. I get it. If you can blame a mother for her child's problems, it makes you feel safer that it can't happen to you or yours. After a year or so of walking this path, which I was still psychologically fighting against, I felt like a total social leper. My self-worth was completely tied to other people's perception of me, and I saw myself the way they did. It was debilitating.

I'd like to say there was one thing that helped, that turned it around, but the truth is that it was a painfully slow process, and one I didn't think I'd survive at times. I took anti-

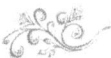

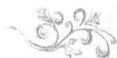

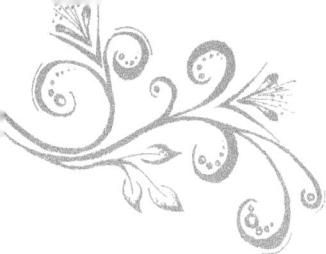

depressants and saw a counsellor; but it was during that phase that I had my most dangerous thoughts. I remember cleaning out my kitchen cupboards with tears rolling down my face, because if I decided I couldn't be here any more I didn't want people to judge me by my messy cupboards.

I left a lot of social activities, and while that might seem like a dangerous thing to do, I believe in the long run it helped remove me from a lot of unhealthy and unhelpful social groups. I understood at this point in my life the definition of "a fair-weather friend".

Ultimately what I appreciate about the process that brought me to where I am now, is the culling of superficial relationships where I constantly battled to feel good enough to be accepted. For the longest time I felt like a failure; that I wasn't as good as the people who were clearly uncomfortable with my current circumstances. Today I can see them for what they are. I know it's not my fault, my weakness, or my deficit. The deficit lies with them.

I do remember though, through all the tears, repeating the mantra "you won't always feel this way". It's not mind-blowing stuff, but I think it helped, and was something to cling to.

I now see those years as a deconstruction of my life, and of who I thought I was. I have no time for pretence now, for the disingenuous small talk of image-conscious people. I surround myself with honest people, who own their

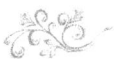

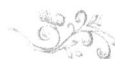

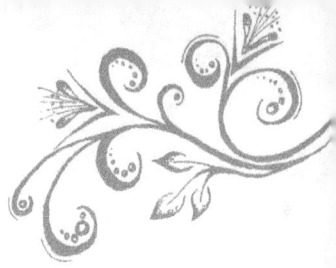

brokenness. I made it through the years when I waited for a phone call to tell me my son was dead, with people, particularly my Christian friends, telling me to be grateful and to give thanks. Stuff that. I've lost my faith, my marriage, a whole ream of friends and associates –but I've gained a more real existence. I have a new daughter, and now a grandchild on the way also. My relationship with my son is solid, and is not tainted by the judgement or expectations of what other people think either of our lives should look like.

I'm sorry if my story hasn't contained much "how to" in terms of coping with depression. I guess in a term that I actually hate, it's more of a testimony that where you are at any one time is not where you are destined to stay. Hardship, like any other experience, is not your final destination, but a valley to pass through. At least that's what it was to me. Surround yourself with the best people. Quality over quantity. Don't suffer people who make you feel less. You are not, never were, and never will be, less than another person. You just have a different journey to travel.

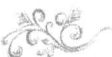

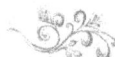

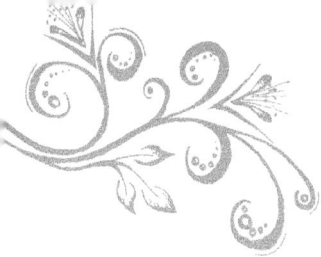

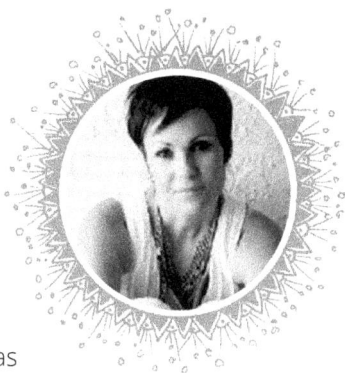

Jacque Opie

I remember asking the universe to crack me open. I remember it like it was yesterday. But it wasn't. It was lifetimes ago. And I forgot. I forgot how numb I was. So numb that tears could not flow. So numb that love could not penetrate my heart. So numb that even the sounds of my crying babies could not move me. And now here I am. On my knees. My heart cracked open. Feeling everything, but wanting numbness.

"All You Need is Love" by John Lennon will never be outdated to me. These are not just words in a song, they are a life motto.

I believe the love I have for myself, and the love that I share with others, is the key to getting myself out of a funk. It doesn't mean that I won't feel like blocking the world out some times; it just means that I recognise I can love myself any time.

When I accept the good and the bad, the pretty and the ugly, the naughty and the nice, within myself, I give myself permission to be, do, have, and experience all of life, not just the fancy bits. Nowadays I love myself enough to realise that ALL of me is okay. Having experienced the self-doubt, self-loathing, and self-criticism for so long, I am much more open to creating more balance in my life, and experiencing self-belief, self-love and self-applause!

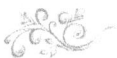

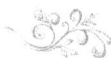

Have you been outside today?

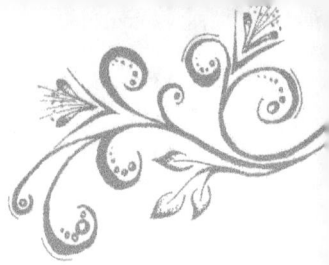

In my darkest hour, I no longer wait for someone to tell me I am amazing. I tell myself. I don't wait until I have achieved something miraculous. I celebrate my little wins. I don't wait until I am on the floor in a heap before I reach out to someone I love and trust to just hold me, feed me, and love me.

Because I know that I am worthy of love, and that I am important in this world. And I know the difference I can make when I am at my peak. There are times when I feel so low that even asking for help is a challenge. I have surrounded myself with people who care for my well-being, and who will look out for me so that even when I can't reach out, they will reach out to me.

Life is like that for me. Yes, I have funk days. And I go on a roller coaster, but at the end of it, I always know I will be OK, because I trust myself. I trust that the challenges I am offered are all within my capability. No one ever told me it was going to be easy, but I know it will be worth it – I am worth it.

And so are you. There is not one person on this earth who is more worthy than you, and not one who is less worthy than you.

Let love flood your soul, your heart, your imagination and your being.

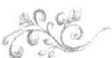

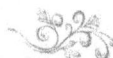

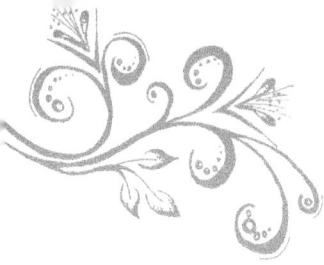

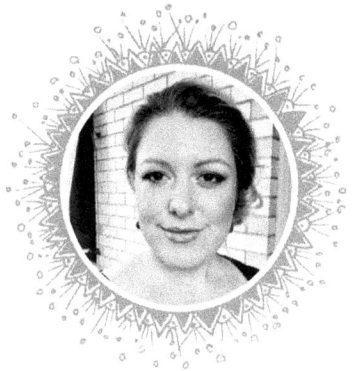

Kate

Ahh...the old funky day. I know it well!

Previously, I would have spent my funk days inside, watching television and numbing-out with food binges. But slowly, I'm getting better at recognising when I'm having one of those days when I just don't feel right, and treating myself with nurturing and understanding.

These days, I find that a walk helps me get out of a funk more than anything else. Often I will go outside for a gentle walk in nature; but it could also be a walk on the treadmill for as little as ten minutes to get my body moving again. I find getting a good sweat-fest going is probably the ultimate in getting those heeby-jeebies out, but any movement works for me.

Another thing I do is try to change my way of thinking about things, and step back from my thought patterns. I live with an anxiety disorder, so often my funk days are characterised by constant obsessive thoughts of things I may have done wrong, or I worry about things that could happen. I try to look objectively at what I'm thinking and to look at things differently, so that I'm not getting bogged down in the "coulda, shoulda, woulda" and "not good enough" narratives that often plague me.

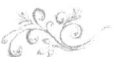

Have you been outside today?

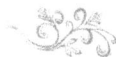

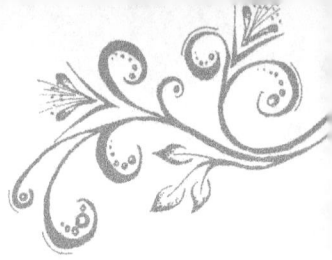

If, for example, I'm obsessing over a mistake I made at work, I try to think of the reasons why I made the mistake and rationalise the implications to make myself feel better.

If I can't do that, sometimes I just have to let myself have a yucky day, with the reassurance that it won't last forever and that the negative feelings will pass.

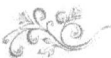

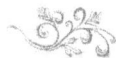

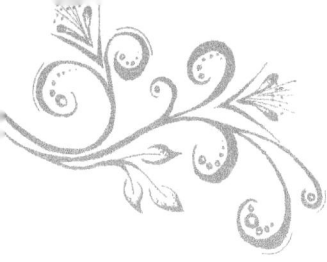

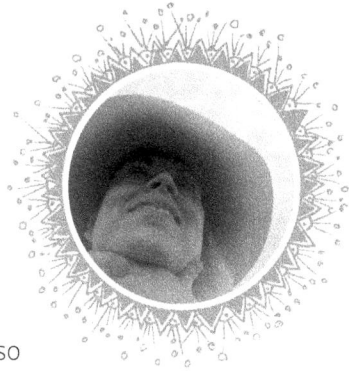

Shani

My experience with mental illness – a bit of feeling depressed here and there but largely anxiety – is so fluid and seamless sometimes that it feels normal. My normal. For instance, I'm very empathetic by nature, and my own emotions are easily swayed by how others around me are feeling. Most of the time this is OK, but sometimes I struggle.

Recently I had some old hurts and experiences coming back around that needed me to feel into – old relationship stuff, fears and judgements. These things were already making it challenging for me to stay clear-headed. So to add on top of that other people's negative experiences or feelings, were extra drips in the bucket that I couldn't handle.

The easiest and usual thing for me to do is avoidance: retreat, isolate and stay away from people. Which will make me feel better initially but can spiral quickly into darkness.

I've learnt that challenging my easiest option is important. In these times, these are the questions I ask myself.

Do I need to be alone? Or do I need to select a positive person to be around?

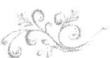

Have you been outside today?

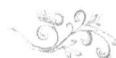

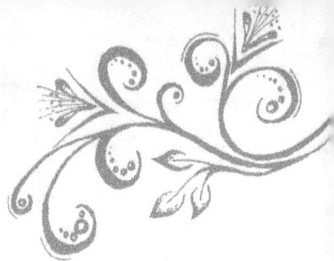

Do I need to be alone at home, closed in and safe? Or can I go to the gym, with headphones in and get endorphins and stress relief, and still be safe?

Is focusing on the problems and rehashing them in my head going to show a solution? Or is sitting, walking, being in nature and clearing my mind a better option?

Is shutting down communication the way? Or can I find a way to "voice" my thoughts via writing or sharing what I'm feeling with someone trusted?

Our natural mechanisms are for safety. Not happiness. I know that the danger is perceived. So I am safe to challenge it.

I've learnt that I can make a big change to my mental health and anxiety by being curious about my feelings, and possibilities, instead of anxious about the outcome.

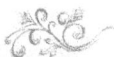

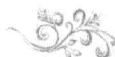

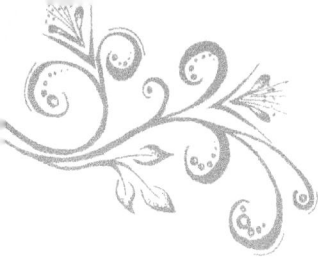

Bel Ryan

Ignite Art Therapies

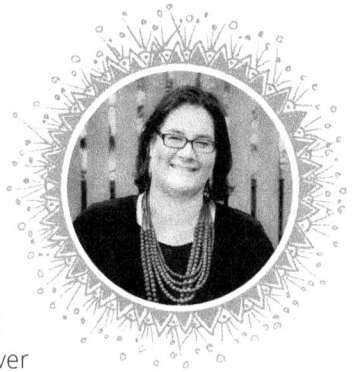

When things get a bit much I just want to enter the cave and never come out. I have learned over time to be aware of the signs of when seeing so many clients starts to impact my own well-being. Once upon a time I would push through, but know that I am a better therapist if I take notice of the signs and actually do something about it.

One of the things that seems to wash away some of the debris is water. Whether it's drinking it, detouring on the way home and jumping in the sea fully clothed, having a shower or bath when I get home, doing aqua aerobics or having some time in a float tank, there is something about the water that cleanses, shifts, equalises and suspends the built-up layers of emotion, trauma, distress that maybe hanging around.

Along with spending some time out in the fresh air or escaping into a movie, water fills my cup so that I can give to others without sucking me dry. This is so important as its very hard to continue on an empty tank.

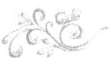

Have you been outside today?

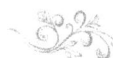

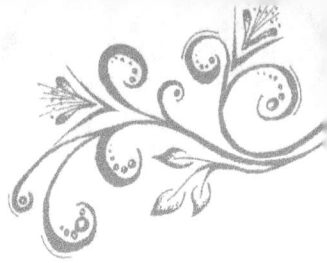

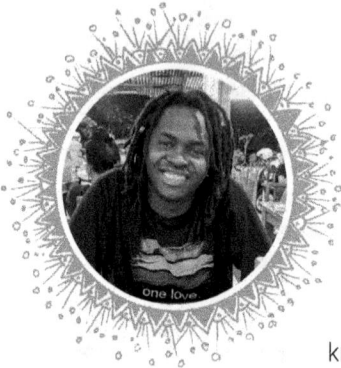

Shanton

When I feel down I really want to go out for a drive, but I don't always know where to go.

In order to feel OK I always want to be by myself. But sometimes a phone call back home to friends and family makes me forget about whatever pressure I am under, or whatever the problem is.

Because I like online auctions, sometimes when I feel upset I just take my computer, look through auctions and see what is the next thing to buy. Some days I like to go to the shop, buy some groceries and start cooking. When I start cooking it's like a meditation to me.

I also like watching news, especially international news, and I love watching documentaries. Taking a nap is also a good thing to do. By the time I wake up after an hour so, I feel fine.

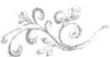

Have you been outside today?

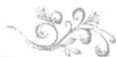

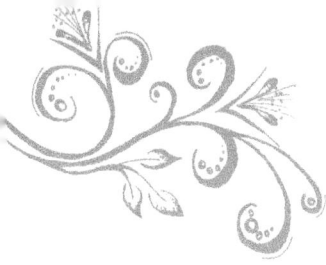

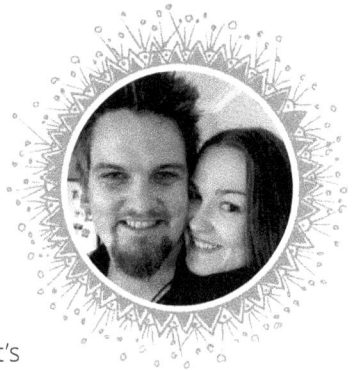

Matt

We all get funky. No, not the kind on the dance floor, the kind where we don't want to do anything. Let's face it, we do. I used to succumb to funks quite frequently.

Being a young single male fresh out of home was, for me at least, not without its tribulations. But it took me a little time to figure out that it was how I dealt with these ruts that defined my resolve and myself. As we all know, motivating yourself to actually move and get out of the funk is the hardest part. But once you realise what works for you, it gets considerably easier.

I'm a person of extremes, and as a result I either needed complete solitude or to lose myself in the company of others. Hence, I have a slightly eclectic mix of funk fixers.

- Meditation. This was a particularly useful one to me. Even if I couldn't achieve full mindfulness, it gave me a moment to reflect on what I was going through and lend some perspective.

- Phone a friend. This was possibly my most frequently used one. I'd call my best mate and have a laugh. Laughter really is the best medicine.

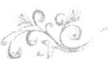

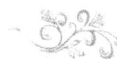

Have you been outside today?

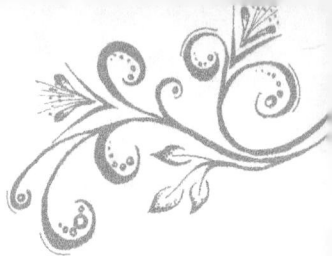

- Go to my local pub. I know, it sounds wrong. But sometimes you gotta go where everybody knows your name. Some firm handshakes, light-hearted banter and a cheeky beer with friends could always lift my spirits.

- Watch a TV show or read a book. I always found that I could easily forget my problems when I was able to immerse myself in another world.

- My girlfriend. These days, this is the only one I need. I can lose myself in her. She never fails to put a smile on my face for a litany of reasons. But she can also firmly realign my perspective, and remind me of what's important.

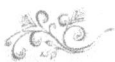

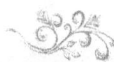

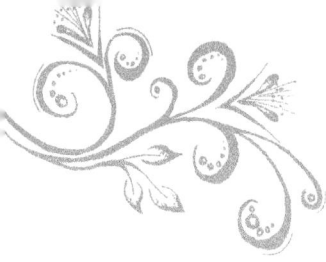

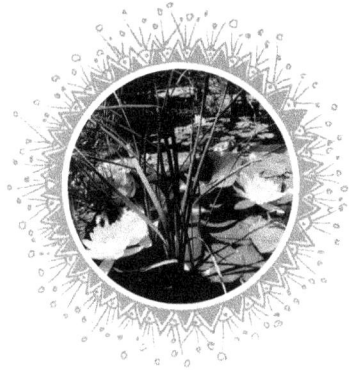

Emmy

There is a very simple equation to kicking the funk out of my day: put myself first.

Easier said than done, right? I am a wife and a mother. My life is looking after my family and the people I love. What happens if your mind and body decide they have had enough and just shut down? It's not fun. It kicks the life out of you. Do you give up and throw in the towel? Of course you don't, it's just a big wake-up call.

When this happens to me it means I need to change things up. I need to ask for help – and accept help too. Sometimes my day is so full of funk that it's virtually impossible to kick.

But I have found looking after myself consistently over a period of time has stopped the feelings being so severe. I have begun to accept that I have these feelings for a reason and it is very important to process them instead of pushing them down. I have stopped feeling so guilty for having time for myself to do things I truly enjoy.

I am not a victim. I am a survivor and will only become stronger and happier the more I take care of me.

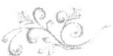 Have you been outside today?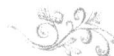

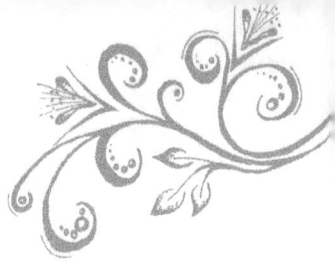

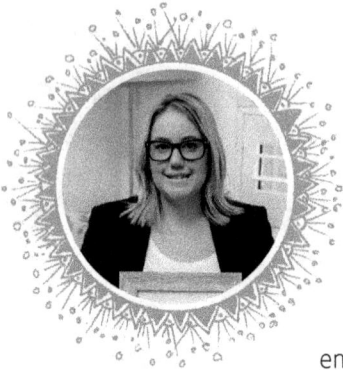

Janelle Lorenzini

www.janellelorenzini.com

Twelve months ago I hit rock bottom emotionally.

I had a good career that I no longer wanted and I was suffering emotional fatigue. I was so exhausted all the time; I just couldn't enjoy life anymore.

In the midst of the darkness inside my head, the negative thoughts that lingered and somewhat consumed me, I said to myself, *There has to be light and this cannot be my life forever.* I wanted to feel better, I wanted to be happier and enjoy life.

Three months before this, I had been seeing a psychologist and she was fabulous; but it came to a point where I now needed to take action and make some changes. I didn't know where I was going, which at the time was unsettling but now I look back, it didn't matter. As long as you keep putting one foot in front of the other, even if you don't know where you are going, it is progress.

I created a Facebook page in March 2016 and started posting positive affirmation images that I found online. This made me accountable daily to search around for beautiful quotes and upload them to my social media. As the months went by, I continued to surround myself with these positive

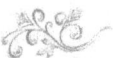 Have you been outside today?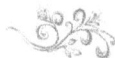

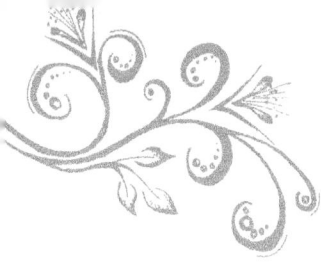

affirmations, say them out loud or to myself and check in and look at them daily. I would also take time to reflect on life, what I enjoyed and could see myself doing for the rest of my life. I would make little notes in a journal of some of my thoughts and as the weeks went on, I would go back and review them.

Over time I noticed that my negative thoughts were fading. I had stopped reflecting for a while and didn't notice the big changes happening inside my head. At the time I was wanting to unplug from social media and give myself a break. Sometimes – too often – I would get stuck in the trap of comparing my life to others' glamorous instagram lives and it made me feel sad and depressed. I couldn't deactivate my account because I relied heavily on the positive affirmations. I wanted so badly a pack of cards that I could put on my desk or in my bathroom to look at every day, physically hold and carry them around with me but I couldn't find any that resonated. That idea led to so many dreams and goals. I decided I wanted to help people who were going through a similar situation.

Fast forward twelve months. I have become an accredited counsellor, created my own inspiration and positive affirmation cards and have just started a Bachelor in Psychological Science (Psychology). Positive affirmations saved my life, they helped me constantly change my thoughts and focus on positive thoughts rather than negative

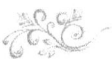

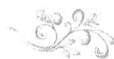

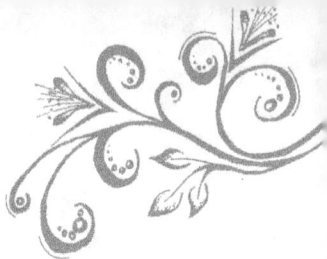

thoughts. The saying "change your thoughts, change your life" is so completely true.

If you are going through a difficult time right now and you don't see that there is a way out, you feel stuck and completely burnt out, remember that it is OK. You will be OK and it will pass – but like anything in life, change starts with you. Be kind to yourself and by that I mean treat yourself through self-love and self-care. Don't put so much pressure on yourself. Keep putting one foot in front of the other, even if you don't know where you are going.

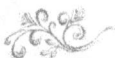

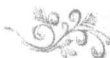

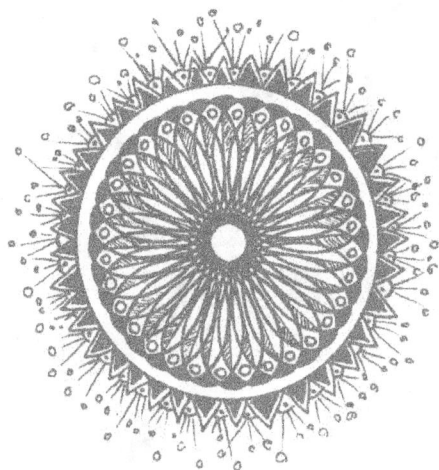

Chapter Seven

Why 108?

A lot of people have asked me why I chose 108 things. First of all, it made you ask the question and got you wondering why I chose that number – so it got your attention!

That actually wasn't the reason why I chose it. 108 is a special number and that's why I chose it but it turned out to have that secondary effect of curiosity. There are so many books titled 99 ways, 101 ways, 100 ways....but I wanted my book to have 108, although in reality there are many more than 108 things in here as you have no doubt found out by now. The core suggestions are 108, but thanks to the valuable contribution of others, it's grown well beyond that.

108 is a significant number for a myriad of reasons, and here are just a few. I could have filled a whole book on this alone, would you believe?

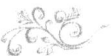 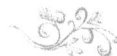

🌼 The number 108 is considered sacred in many Eastern religions and traditions, such as Hinduism, Buddhism, Jainism, Sikhism and connected yoga and dharma based practices.

🌼 The pre-historic monument Stonehenge is 108 feet in diameter.

🌼 The number 108 is known to refer to spiritual completion, and it is no surprise that the early Vedic sages were renowned mathematicians and in fact invented our number system.

🌼 The distance between the Earth and the Sun is 108 times the diameter of the Sun. The diameter of the Sun is 108 times the diameter of the Earth. The distance between the Earth and Moon is 108 times the diameter of the Moon. The universe is made up of 108 elements according to ancient texts. (The current periodic table claims a few more than 108.)

🌼 There are 12 constellations and nine arc segments: 9 x 12 = 108.

🌼 One of the major interpretations of the number 108 is the number of the 12 zodiac signs multiplied with nine planets in the zodiac: 9 x 12 = 108.

🌼 The first manned space flight lasted 108 minutes.

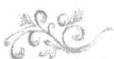 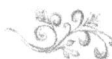

🏵 Hindu deities have 108 names, while in Gaudiya Vaishnavism, there are 108 gopis of Vrindavan. Recital of these names, often accompanied by the counting of the 108-beaded mala, is considered sacred and often done during religious ceremonies.

🏵 The Buddhist rosary, which inspired the rosary of Muslims, then – via the Crusades – that of Catholic Christians, is constituted of 108 fragments of distinctive different human skulls.

🏵 The holy writings for Tibetans are made up of 108 sacred books.

🏵 The Vedanta, according to the Hinduism tradition, recognises 108 authentic doctrines (Upanishad) aiming to approach the truth and to destroy Ignorance.

🏵 In Jain, there is a tradition that there are 108 virtues.

🏵 There are 54 letters in the Sanskrit alphabet. Each has masculine and feminine, shiva and shakti: 54 times 2 is 108.

🏵 Lankavatara Sutra ancient teachings refer repeatedly to many temples with 108 steps.

🏵 In Tibetan Buddhism it is believed that there are 108 sins or 108 delusions of the mind.

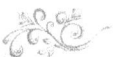

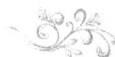

⚙ According to Chinese and Indian martial arts, Marma Adi and Ayurveda, there are 108 pressure points in a human body.

⚙ There are 108 lords of the Tao according to Taoism.

⚙ There are 108 columns of the temple of Ourga.

⚙ Phnom Bakheng in Angkor has 108 towers.

⚙ According to yogic tradition, there are 108 sacred sites throughout India. There are 108 marma points or sacred places of the body.

⚙ There are 108 stitches on a baseball.

⚙ The sum of "the numbers" in the TV show *Lost* is 108 (4, 8, 15, 16, 23, and 42). It is also the number of minutes within which these numbers must be entered into the computer and the button must be pushed. Oceanic 6 spent 108 days on the island.

⚙ There are 108 cards in an Uno deck.

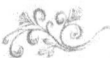 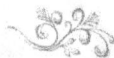

Acknowledgements

I am one of those people who actually reads acknowledgements in books. I find them heart-warming and interesting, despite the fact that I don't know any of the people mentioned. As a writer, or any kind of artist, it's incredibly important to acknowledge the people who have our backs and are with us through thick and thin. I hope you take the time to read mine, as this book would definitely not have been possible without the support and input of these amazing people.

Angela, Laura, Jamie, Erica, Meekehleh, Noma, Elmina, Bron, Aylee, Waratah, Leah, Jacque, Kate, Shani, Bel, Matt, Emmy, Janelle and Shanton; thank you from the bottom of my heart for sharing your stories with such honesty and courage. This book changed completely because of all of you. Words cannot express my gratitude.

Aylee, you come into a category all of your own. You are my soul sister, my best friend, my lifeline, my shoulder, my ear and my "move a body" friend. No matter how funky I am or what happens, you are there for me, always. You also have impeccable taste and helped the cover of this book to be the masterpiece that it is. I love you more than words.

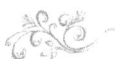 Have you been outside today?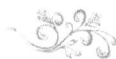

Jamie, my writing buddy and non-judgemental listening ear. Thank you for your input, your creativity and ideas on so many aspects of this book. Thank you for always being available when I need help or a question answered. I am so excited that we are publishing our books at the same time and I look forward to more of the journey with you. And yes, we are all just walking each other home.

Emma, your artistic talents are nothing short of remarkable. Your beautiful mandalas have brought this book to life and the love and attention to detail you put into drawing them shines through. Thank you my friend.

My family – my amazing sons Josh and Matt, and my gorgeous grandchildren Ella and Jake – you make me proud every single day. I love you all more than words and I am so honoured to be your mum and grandma.

Jess, you are such a talented photographer with a wonderful eye for catching incredible moments of beauty. I am so proud to have your photo of me on this book.

Mum, you are by far the most inspiring, courageous and incredible woman I've ever known. I am so grateful to have had you as a mother, teacher, inspiration, role model and constant unwavering source of unconditional love and support.

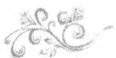

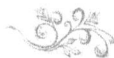

And finally Shanton, my loving husband, best friend and biggest fan. You, my love, have taught me what true freedom and love are. You have stood by my side from day one and encouraged me to be all that I am and inspired me to step up and follow my dreams. I love you with all of my heart.

With so much love and gratitude,

Rae-Anne ☺ xx

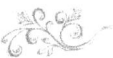
Have you been outside today?
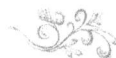

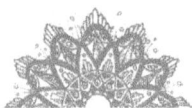

"Real isn't how you are made," said the Skin Horse. "It's a thing that happens to you. When a child loves you for a long, long time, not just to play with, but REALLY loves you, then you become Real."

"Does it hurt?" asked the Rabbit.

"Sometimes," said the Skin Horse, for he was always truthful. "When you are Real you don't mind being hurt."

"Does it happen all at once, like being wound up," he asked, "or bit by bit?"

"It doesn't happen all at once," said the Skin Horse. "You become. It takes a long time. That's why it doesn't happen often to people who break easily, or have sharp edges, or who have to be carefully kept. Generally, by the time you are Real, most of your hair has been loved off, and your eyes drop out and you get loose in the joints and very shabby. But these things don't matter at all, because once you are Real you can't be ugly, except to people who don't understand."

– Margery Williams, The Velveteen Rabbit

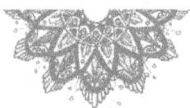

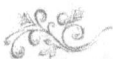

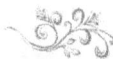

Have you been outside today?

www.ingramcontent.com/pod-product-compliance
Lightning Source LLC
Chambersburg PA
CBHW050123280326
41933CB00010B/1223